The Public Health and The NHS
your questions answered

Norman Vetter

RADCLIFFE MEDICAL PRESS

© 1998 Norman Vetter

Radcliffe Medical Press Ltd
18 Marcham Road, Abingdon, Oxon OX14 1AA, UK

British Library Cataloguing in Publication Data

A catalogue record for this book is available from the British Library.

ISBN 1 85775 299 6

Typeset by Advance Typesetting Ltd, Oxon
Printed and bound by Biddles Ltd, Guildford and King's Lynn

Contents

Acknowledgements   iv

1   Problems of health services   1

2   The 1940s: origins of the NHS and early responses   20

3   The 1950s and 1960s: catching up on new developments   36

4   The 1970s: reorganization begins   49

5   The 1980s: how many reorganizations do you want?   61

6   The 1990s: the market will provide, then stopped providing   75

7   The 2000s   94

8   Conclusion: has it worked?   117

References   124

Index   128

Acknowledgements

I acknowledge the help of Diane Richards and Anna Ledgard in the preparation of this book. I also thank my secretaries, Julia Hodgson and Ann Bushell for word processing much of it.

1

Problems of health services

▲ 1 What is this book about?

My main idea in writing this book is to suggest that health services exist 'in place of fear', in Aneurin Bevan's phrase, and that they should be judged according to that criterion. They are not good at reducing deaths or disability. Health services do save some lives and prevent some disability, but the most efficient means of doing this in the health service is by vaccination and immunization. These are regarded as a peripheral, low status part of any service. So the core of the organization has a marginal effect on deaths and disability, virtually non-existent when compared with the sweeping effects of environmental and personal changes, especially those which result from people across the board becoming better off financially.

I have tried to prove this idea using the UK National Health Service (NHS) as an example. This has the advantage of having a finite beginning on 7 July 1948 when sweeping changes were made to the way that health services were provided for the whole population. It is therefore possible to examine what happened when everyone in the country was, for the first time, allowed free access to high quality health services. The change relieved many people of fear but had little effect upon death or disability rates. I go on to suggest that if relieving fear is what the NHS does best we should change some of the things we do in future.

▲ 2 What is the evidence that the NHS has virtually no effect on deaths or disability?

The setting up of the NHS in 1948 was intended to reduce deaths and disability. Figure 1.1 shows data on deaths in infants from the turn of the century onwards. It can be seen that the infant mortality rate has fallen steadily since 1900, with no marked variation, except for during the Second World War. The NHS does not seem to have resulted in any obvious change in a steadily improving rate. My

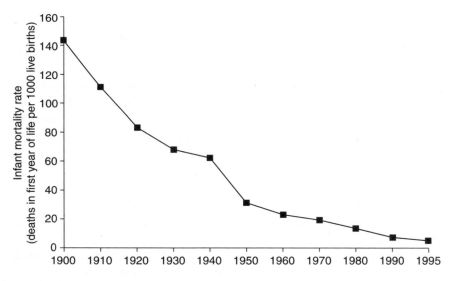

Figure 1.1: Infant mortality rate: UK.

point is not that the NHS had no effect, we do not know what would have happened without it, simply that the major change in the organization of the health service in 1948 had, at most, a minor effect, not discernible at a national level.

Similar figures for life expectancy at birth and life expectancy at age 65 show no unusual improvement due to the advent of the NHS. Indeed life expectancy at birth appears to decelerate after the 1940s, though it does continue to rise (Figures 1.2 and 1.3).

Data on disability over this period are much more difficult to find. Data on incapacity for work have been available since the 1950s (Figure 1.4) and show that incapacity has steadily increased while mortality has been decreasing. The picture is not clear because a large number of people are marginally incapacitated. When unemployment rises they tend to be thrown out of the labour market more rapidly than able-bodied people. Changes in incapacity rates may therefore reflect unemployment rather than any NHS effect. Other issues swamp any effect that the NHS may have.

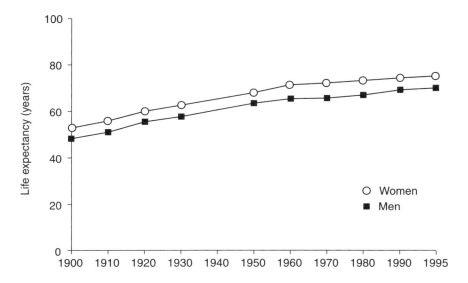

Figure 1.2: Life expectancy at birth: England and Wales.

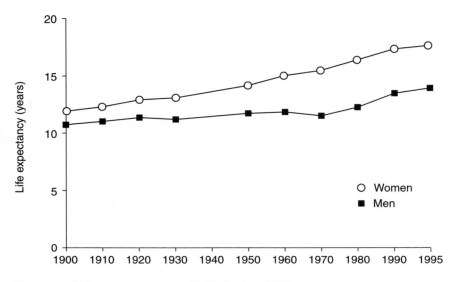

Figure 1.3: Life expectancy at age 65: England and Wales.

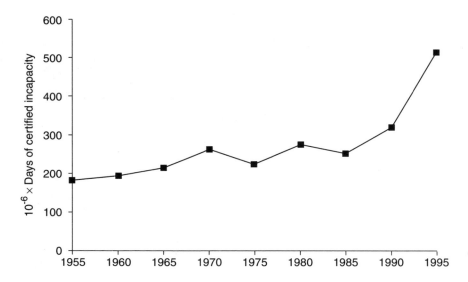

Figure 1.4: Days of certified incapacity: men.

Figures 1.1–1.4 bear out my thesis through this book, that death and disability rates are little, if at all, influenced by health services, even such a major improvement as making all health care free for all.

▲ 3 What is wrong with trying to reduce death and disability?

It is unlikely that the NHS or any other health service in developed countries will have a great effect on death or disability. Virtually all of the effort expended within the NHS, for example, is to treat people who are at a late stage of the disease process which can only be slightly modified in terms of their future death and disability. Professionals increasingly battle to bring about marginal improvements in people with increasingly severe disease. The cost of this rises year on year with little effect upon the patients' outcomes. The law of diminishing returns has set in with a vengeance in medicine. Professionals can ignore this because they have not been aware of the figures. In future with better information and more emphasis upon measuring effectiveness, this 'head in the sand' approach will no longer be possible.

At present the relationship between health professionals and patients is taken up with trying to persuade patients that most treatment is extremely effective in terms of death and disability avoided. This is not true and most professionals know it is not. The relationship is therefore a con. To make things worse, very few professionals are good at lying so that patients constantly suspect that they are being kept in the dark about the real state of affairs. However patients are becoming more knowledgeable about the issues around health and disease and increasingly skilled at seeing through the subterfuges thrown up by their professional staff.

In the past, health care staff suffered from problems, which might have been an excuse for their behaviour. They often did not know the right way to approach a problem themselves because there was either no consensus, or there were a number of consensuses, about the best way to treat it. They would use the method they had been taught by their own teacher and often believed this to be correct, without evidence. There are no excuses for this any more. The number of guidelines, protocols and evidence-based tracts that exist and are freely available to professionals is legion. In the rare cases where there is no consensus, the best way to relieve the fear of the patients must be to come clean and try to work through the problem together. There is still often nothing that medicine can offer except palliation by the time a patient goes to their doctor.

▲ 4 What evidence is there that reducing deaths and disabilities is the main aim of the NHS?

I have said that, at present, the people running the NHS regard its main function as reducing death and disabilities, with relieving fear a secondary or tertiary issue. I need to defend that statement. In 1991 the government of the day produced a document which was welcomed throughout the NHS as the first national strategy for England.[1] This contained a large number of targets for the health service over the following years. Virtually all of them were about reducing deaths or disability. A more recent example, which shows the importance placed on these measures, has been the Labour government's suggestion that the outcomes of medical care should be made available to the general public, so that hospitals can be compared, the good and the bad. They have suggested that the measures should be similar to those used in Scotland for a number of years. Most are related to death rates for different diseases so that different hospitals and health authorities may be compared.

It is obvious that a specialist unit with significantly high death or disability rates should have their figures examined in some detail in case poor techniques may be causing them. Professionals who are causing more harm than good obviously need to be removed from the care of patients. This is different from judging the effectiveness of health services according to such criteria in large populations.

▲ 5 Why 'in place of fear'?

Aneurin Bevan wrote *In Place of Fear* in the early 1960s. This appears to have been the central tenet of his belief in the NHS. Its aim was to remove fear at a number of levels:

- fear of death and disease and its effects
- fear of not being able to afford treatment
- fear that the cost of treatment would bring families near to destitution in order to meet the bills.

This last fear is well understood in the present day USA by those who are not adequately covered by health insurance.

My contention is that the primary function of the NHS is still, nearly 50 years later, to relieve fear. However, if relieving fear is to be the main function there are a number of important consequences (Box 1.1), some of which may not be immediately obvious.

Doctors and nurses have concentrated on reducing deaths and disability, often called 'hard outcomes' in health service jargon. This has resulted in a mechanistic approach to health care, aimed at reducing the physical effects of disease as a priority. Relieving fear has had a lesser priority. It has been assumed, as far as it has been thought of at all, that the confidence of the professionals in their own power to defeat death and disability will brush off on patients, relieving their fear. Professionals have therefore spent their time trying to persuade their patients of their infallibility, not in trying to relieve fear by explanation of the true situation. This does not work. The frustration patients feel at the lack of true understanding they get from their doctors and nurses grows continuously.

Box 1.1 If the main function of the health service is to relieve fear

Many of the things carried out in the name of the health service are not effective therefore:

- We must stop carrying out these functions.
- Patient confidence will be kept if they understand why some common procedures are discontinued and are guaranteed relief from serious symptoms.
- This will be undermined if the health service professionals lie to themselves or their patients about the effectiveness of ineffective treatment.

This in turn has consequences:

- Patients must not be led to expect the impossible.
- Patients must clearly be told what the health service can, and cannot, do.
- Health authorities have a duty to give information about health, disease and the health service to the population.

To relieve fear effectively doctors and nurses need to include their doubts and concerns about the disease and the treatment, as well as the positive aspects of the approach they are taking. This changes the approach from one of patient versus professional to one of patient and professional versus the disease.

▲ 6 How should we relieve fear in the NHS?

In health services three main problems predominate which exacerbate fear for patients: pain, ignorance and poverty. The NHS, while alleviating the fear of not being able to afford treatment has been slow to establish ways of dealing with pain and ignorance.

▲ 7 How well has the NHS tried to relieve fear by the treatment of pain?

The treatment of pain has been such a problem within the NHS that it has now become a specialty of its own. The development of a specialty to cover an area of health is a sign that the experts in that field are not happy with the way it is being carried out, and pain care is no exception. Many researchers over the years have shown that our treatment of patients in pain is inadequate. In my early days in medicine, in the late 1960s, patients waiting to have an operation to relieve pain from their peptic ulcers were often left for a while. It was suggested that this would reduce the proportion of patients who continued to complain of symptoms, after their operation. The wait was suggested so that they would 'earn' their operation and that the reduction of symptoms would be such that they would put up with the minor inconveniences of the remaining side effects of the operation.

A colleague caused a considerable stir in the specialty by suggesting that some people did well, some did not and it was nothing to do with the amount of pain that they had endured prior to the treatment. She showed that patients did well or badly according to their personality, not the degree of their symptoms, and that operating early or late made no difference to how well they did.

▲ 8 How well has the NHS tried to relieve fear by removing ignorance?

Maintaining patients' ignorance is endemic in many health services, but especially so in the NHS. This is found at all levels. The commonest complaint that patients have about their care is that they do not understand what is going on.[2] At its most extreme, some patients, if they have not received a particular service, remain unaware of its existence. This was found to be the case when questioning people about community services.[3] People aged 70 and over were asked about services they were likely to, or had already, received. Less than half of them were aware of the work of common services, such as sheltered housing, the incontinence laundry service and bath attendants. Researchers have shown that levels of demand for services are inversely related to the disability of the recipients of the service.[4] This is a 'catch 22' situation where those most in need of a service are least likely to know about it.

A lovely BMA pamphlet[5] published in 1977 would be considered politically incorrect now but still seems to sum up the approach of health care workers to pregnant women:

… you are going to have to answer a lot of questions and be the subject of a lot of examinations. Never worry about any of these. They are necessary, they are in the interests of your baby and yourself, and none of them will ever hurt you.

At a population level we are a secretive society in the UK. An example of this came to me earlier this year. I published widely some data about waiting times for individual consultants in Wales, which were already available on the Internet. I received a number of complaints that surgeons should be mentioned by name. This protest was only a little abated when I explained that the average 12-year old could easily get hold of the data on the Internet. The data were, shortly afterwards, removed from open.gov, the government's Internet site.

▲ 9 Is relieving fear the only thing the NHS could or should do?

The NHS does a large number of other things by existing. Perhaps the most important is that it provides employment for about a million people in the UK. It may be argued that any form of health service would do the same, but the centralized nature of the NHS has meant that salaries and conditions of service have been kept at a similar level throughout the country. The NHS as a single entity needs a huge number of staff to run it. In its early days these needs were impossible to fulfil except by importing large numbers of doctors and nurses from what were then the colonies. Great numbers of doctors who had qualified in India and Pakistan came to the UK, initially to obtain post-graduate training. Many stayed on after training and filled posts in the fast-expanding NHS. It has been suggested that the cost to these developing countries of losing their doctors to the UK was many times more than the foreign aid which we provided for them. Nurses came in numbers from the West Indies and again must have considerably drained the economies of those countries in their loss of trained staff.

The NHS has therefore given stable employment to a large number of people, which in itself has a direct effect on health. A colleague, Nigel Moss, produced one of the most direct measures of this by showing a direct relationship between hospital admission and unemployment in the electoral wards of Cardiff (Figure 1.5). The figure shows the relationship between the two.

There is a lot of evidence which shows how rapidly a patient's psychological state improves when they get back to work after different diseases. One of the most widely researched is the beneficial effect of getting back to work after a heart attack.[6] Work and health are therefore closely interrelated.

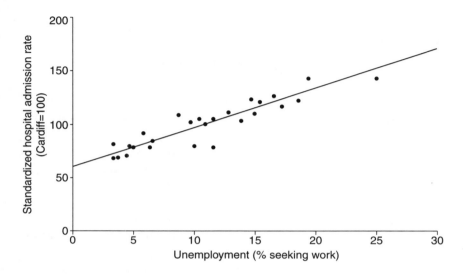

Figure 1.5: Unemployment and admissions to hospital by electoral ward for Cardiff in 1993.

▲ 10 What else does the NHS do that helps the country?

The NHS does many other things that are of help to the country. It has an important training function, from post-graduate training for doctors, nurses and therapists to training for theatre technicians. In addition, a great deal of training in general skills is carried on. The NHS employs large numbers of administrative, finance, personnel and secretarial staff. A great deal of expertise goes into the processing of data.

The health service data, on disease and disability, are used by many other groups, especially the local authority planning and housing departments, as well as groups interested in transport and road development. Pure medical research is, theoretically, carried out by the research councils and charitable trusts, but inevitably much support is given by the NHS, if only by allowing ready access to large numbers of patients.

▲ 11 Does the NHS have no effect upon health?

Curiously, there is little agreement about what is meant by health so that before we can agree on what affects it, we need to decide what it is. A healthy person can be thought of as someone who looks happy. Interestingly, it has been suggested that happiness is an abnormal psychological state, an illness. Richard Bentall has argued that happiness meets all of the criteria for a psychiatric disorder. It is statistically abnormal and consists of a cluster of symptoms, which are usually present. There is some evidence that it reflects abnormal functioning of the central nervous system and is associated with a lack of contact with reality. He suggests that the term happiness be replaced by the more formal psychiatric description 'major affective disorder, pleasant type'.[7]

A wide range of things markedly affects the health of individuals. An attempt has been made by Lalonde to classify these (Box 1.2); he suggested that there were four main elements to health.

These factors are not in order of importance, except that all observers agree that health care services, including the NHS, are the least important. Some people even go so far as to say that they are irrelevant. It is certainly difficult to find evidence that suggests that health services have a measurable impact on health or disease in developed countries. There is some evidence from developing countries which suggests that factors other than the wealth of the country, probably the organization of the health and other welfare services, may have an effect.

Work has been carried out to compare countries such as China, Sri Lanka and Kerala State in India which have gross national products (GNPs) per head of about $300 with Saudi Arabia which

---

Box 1.2 What affects the health of individuals?

- **Human biology:** genetic inheritance, the process of ageing and the robustness of our 'body systems'.
- **The environment:** those factors related to health, external to the person and over which the individual has little or no control, e.g. adequacy of sanitation, water supply, atmospheric pollution, radiation.
- **Lifestyle:** the aggregation of decisions by individuals that affect their health and over which they have ostensibly some control, e.g. smoking, diet. It includes the factor known to have greatest influence on an individual's health over which there is some possibility of change; their personal wealth.
- **Health care services:** quantity, quality and access to health care.

---

has a GNP per head of \$12 200, close to that of the USA. The life expectancy in the former countries was 65 years, in Saudi Arabia 56. The main factors which seemed to control these contrary figures were good primary health care and a good primary educational system.[8]

In developed countries, infectious diseases can be largely controlled with a basic health service. The common non-infectious diseases are mainly of unknown cause so that little can be done to prevent them directly. Health services in developed countries therefore mainly end up trying to salvage people who are extremely ill at a relatively late stage of their disease. A few diseases could be prevented because they are closely related to reversible factors, notably lung cancer and other diseases related to smoking. Even in these diseases our society has found it impossible greatly to reduce the proportion of people who smoke, and has made few serious attempts to do so. This makes the knowledge that smoking is related to a high likelihood of disease useless for all practical purposes. For example, young women, the fittest group in most developed societies are increasing their smoking year on year.

There appears to be a preference in the developed world, the NHS in particular, for hitting our heads against brick walls.

▲ 12 If health services do not avoid death and disability, what does?

Factors that are most closely related to health in developed countries are mainly related to wealth. There is a close relationship between health measures and the average wealth of the population. Figure 1.6 shows data for the UK comparing the wealth of the country, measured as the gross domestic product, with the infant mortality rate.

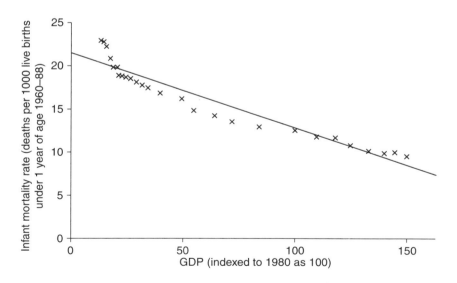

Figure 1.6: Relationship in the UK between infant mortality rate and gross domestic product.

It can be seen that they are very closely related over the period in question, the 1960s to the 1980s.

Infant mortality rate is generally agreed to be the best single indicator of the health of a country, although others do exist. Another measure that we can use is life expectancy. Infant mortality rate gives some useful information about the beginning of life. A measure, which is useful at the end of life, is life expectancy at age 65. Life expectancy at younger ages tends to be slow to show the impact of changes. Figure 1.7 shows changes in life expectancy at age 65 for women by gross domestic product for the UK over the same period. It can be seen that there is a very clear relationship between the two, suggesting that the wealth of the country is also closely allied to longevity.

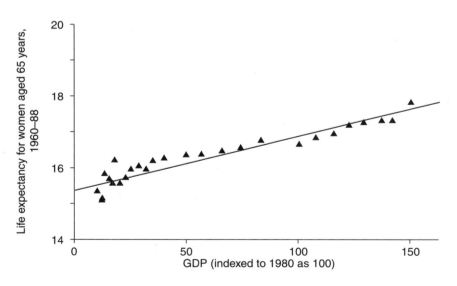

Figure 1.7: Relationship in the UK between life expectancy (women aged 65) and gross domestic product.

▲ 13 Why do those who need it most get least from health services? – the inverse care law

Even if doctors are doing no harm, they may not be doing as much good as they might if they concentrate on the wrong patients. This is Dr Julian Tudor Hart's famous inverse care law: 'The availability of good medical care tends to vary inversely with the need for it in the population served'.[9] This is one of the central problems of poor people receiving health care, even in a health service free at the point of care. A good example of this is for immunization against childhood infectious diseases, where poorer people are more likely to suffer serious consequences of the infectious diseases and also less likely to take up immunization against them.

The reasons for this are due to a wide range of different things (Box 1.3).

Different approaches are needed for poor communities compared with more affluent communities. It has been suggested that more proactive, stronger primary care services are needed to overcome travel problems and more self-help groups can overcome the suspicion derived from cultural problems.

Box 1.3 Reasons for inverse care law

Reasons for greater incidence of disease in poorer people
- Poor environment: poor housing, more pollution in atmosphere, poor work environment, e.g. noisy, polluted atmosphere.
- Lifestyle factors: smoking, less nutritious food, especially fresh fruit and vegetables, excessive drinking more likely.
- Travel problems: difficulty getting to supermarkets and cheaper food.

Box 1.3 *continued*

Reasons for lower uptake of health and social services
- Poorer provision of services, e.g. general practitioners of poorer quality, less proactive than in well-to-do areas.
- Travel problems: inability to get to centralized GP services.
- Inability to work the system, lack of telephones to get GP appointments.
- Cultural factors: doctors, teachers find it easier to understand problems of similar professionals.

▲ 14 Why do we have health services at all?

Developed countries have established a body of knowledge which, superficially at any rate, is standardized in terms of how to describe severe illness. The World Health Organization codifies the illnesses that people suffer in the International Classification of Diseases. This describes diseases in terms of the symptoms suffered by the patient and the results of tests carried out by health staff. They are accepted in all of the developed countries of the world. The diagnostic descriptions contained in the international classification led to another body of knowledge, also quite well codified between different countries on the treatment of each diagnostic tag and its likely outcome.

In developed countries the way health services approach the diagnosis, treatment and care for their patients in practice is therefore surprisingly uniform. In virtually all developed countries there are staff who concentrate on seeing patients when they first feel unwell, often called primary care staff, and those who are expert at the most serious illnesses which require special expertise. The primary care staff have a particularly difficult function, that of deciding if a patient is really ill or whether they are simply angling for the privileges, such as being off work, that illness brings. Another difficulty is when a patient truly believes themself to be ill but the health staff cannot find a problem that fits into the model of illness. This sorting out process can cause considerable anguish for patients and staff.

This description of the uniformity of what is sometimes termed 'western' medicine can be exaggerated. It has been estimated, for instance, that, in the USA in 1990, 425 million visits were made to a range of alternative, unconventional therapists compared with 388 visits to primary care physicians.[10] Expenditure in that year on alternative therapies was $13.7 billion.

2

The 1940s: origins of the NHS and early responses

▲ 15 What sort of treatment was available for patients in the 1940s?

William Silverman tells a story about his professor of pharmacology in 1939. Holding up a bottle of the first sulphonamide, Prontosil, the precursor of a rush of very effective anti-bacterial agents he said: 'Gentlemen, this will work. And do you know why it will work. Because it's red!'[11]

Silverman mentions that this rejection of new ideas was probably a long-standing reaction to the horrors of the over-interventionist 18th and first half of the 19th century where dangerous interventions, such as bleeding and purging, vied with each other to kill off the patient more quickly. The mid 19th century saw the development of numerical methods of comparing results of treatment with no treatment. This made it obvious to the professionals that, beyond the anecdote, their treatment was often worse than useless.

The emphasis within medicine was diagnosis, but following that intervention was often limited to relieving symptoms. The mid to late 1940s saw the rapid development of a number of anti-microbial medicines, which, for the first time, were effective at treating life-threatening infectious diseases.

▲ 16 Why did we have an NHS?

The NHS grew, with the welfare state in general, from an aspiration to have a better life after the Second World War. From the government's point of view this was undoubtedly used as a means of maintaining morale during the fighting. An important component of the government was the Ministry of Reconstruction, which was given the task of planning the way that the country would return to normal when the war was over. For many people returning to the normal life as they had known it in the 1930s was not an especially pleasant prospect. The war for many people, despite the obvious dangers and privations, was exciting and worthwhile. The promises for a new 'welfare state' made during the war were so powerful that the electorate voted Labour into power, as the party the electorate believed would carry out the promises. The strength of this hope was such that even Churchill, the figurehead of the government during the war and a popular hero, lost his position as Prime Minister.

The war also drew together people from different social groups who had had little contact before the war. Such upheavals as sending working class evacuees from the inner cities to middle class families in the country to escape the bombing, while at the same time sending middle class city children to poor families in the country, shocked the country with the awareness of the dreadful physical, educational and social state of the poor. It is said that the blitz, opening up the flats and houses of the poor in the East End of London to public gaze, gave a similar impetus to new house building.

The health services desperately needed reorganizing. The hospital services in particular were in a mess, with two main groups of hospitals competing with each other for custom. These were the voluntary hospitals, originally set up by rich benefactors, and the local authority hospitals. The voluntary hospitals had been very short of money until payments under the Emergency Medical Service for servicemen and other people affected by the war helped them to survive. The voluntary and local authority hospitals were therefore glad of a place in the framework of the health services, without the competitiveness that had been growing up between them.

▲ 17 How did people pay for health services before the NHS?

Concerns about providing health care, especially to poor people, had grown over many years until, in 1911, David Lloyd George introduced a bill to provide compulsory National Insurance for manual workers with incomes below £160 per annum. General practitioner (GP) services were paid for by the 'ninepence for fourpence' system where the state paid two pence, the employer three pence and the employee four pence a week to the National Health Insurance scheme. Over 40% of the adult population was covered by this scheme by the late 1930s. Most GPs took some part in the scheme as 'panel doctors'. The approved societies who ran the schemes often offered extra cover for dentistry, spectacles, and sometimes hospital care, although this last was rare. Non-earners were not covered. School children and the poor could get free treatment if they failed the 'family means test'.

Hospital treatment at the voluntary hospitals was often free to those who could not afford to pay. The 1911 Act did not affect hospitals, although some central government funds were provided for setting up TB sanatoriums. The societies administering the system were, however, authorized to make grants to voluntary hospitals, thus enabling some relatively poor working people to make use of them.

▲ 18 What did people do before the NHS for visiting a GP?

The 'ninepence for fourpence' system gave people three main benefits: cash for any period of incapacity which made them unable to work, the costs of GP care and drug costs. The patients had no freedom of choice about which doctor they would see, neither were doctors involved in the administration of the Act.

GPs were mainly single-handed, with only their wife answering queries about the whereabouts of her husband. Receptionists were very rare and most GPs worked from their own homes. Poor patients, seen on the 'panel' system would often be seen at lock-up surgeries and private patients in the GP's own home. Some GPs waived their fees for poor people, but in poor areas GPs themselves were not well off.

▲ 19 How did hospitals develop?

For many years hospitals had been divided, as mentioned above, into two main types: the hospitals run by the local authorities, some of which were the descendants of the Poor Law hospitals within the workhouses, and the voluntary hospitals. These last were originally set up by rich benefactors, especially in the 18th and 19th centuries, and were often very beautiful buildings. Boards of Governors ran them.

Between the wars, a number of official committees encouraged ideas for establishing the existing two hospital systems on a sounder footing, particularly because of the financial crises regularly facing the voluntary hospitals. Most of the suggested reforms were strongly resisted by the medical profession, because they feared state control. A Royal Commission in 1926 first suggested that the only way for the majority of the population to be able to enjoy costly medical services would be to pay for the services through general public funds, that is by taxation.

The demands on hospitals by casualties during the Second World War pinpointed the awkwardness of the system, especially the voluntary hospitals. During the war, voluntary hospitals were well paid for their beds but, despite this, they still tried to reject long-term and elderly patients, supposedly in order to have as many emergency beds available as possible. The Emergency Medical Service, set up for the treatment of war casualties, employed hospital doctors on a full-time salaried basis.

These wartime changes were partial and short-term but they changed public attitudes towards hospital care so that a large-scale reorganization of the existing services was inevitable. It has been argued that the Second World War saved the voluntary hospitals from financial disaster but it also emphasized the great financial problems that they had and finally led to them being integrated with the local authority hospitals into the NHS.

▲ 20 How did people receive hospital care before the NHS?

After the First World War, hospitals had become increasingly more orientated towards being specialist consultation centres, although the outpatient departments continued to act as dispensaries for poor people and GPs still did some specialist work in areas that were short of manpower, such as anaesthetics and obstetrics. GPs had some beds for patients in their cottage hospitals and nursing homes. The increasing financial pressure on the voluntary hospitals caused them to introduce charges, even for poor people, and a few pay bed wards for middle class patients. Charges consisted of a contribution from patients according to a means test.

The public, local authority run, hospitals attempted to care for all of the patients in their catchment area. They provided three-quarters of the hospital beds although, because these patients tended to have chronic diseases and to be more elderly, they were in hospital for much longer periods than those in the voluntary hospitals. The beds therefore probably served a considerably smaller proportion of the people who needed care. The finance for the public hospitals was mainly from the local councils and grants from central government. Unlike the voluntary hospitals, all of the staff were paid. Public hospitals, in contrast with the voluntary hospitals, treated chronic and elderly patients, people with infectious diseases, maternity and mental cases. The voluntary hospitals were resistant to taking such people and concentrated on acute and short-term care for general medical and surgical patients. This division has remained as a partition between the posh and not-so-posh parts of medical care to this day.

▲ 21 How did the idea of the NHS develop?

In 1933, the Socialist Medical Association first suggested the provision of a free, tax-supported service on a universal basis with doctors working on full-time salaries and with full professional freedom. The service was to be organized around health centres for outpatient care and large general hospitals for institutional care. The administration was to be looked after by local authorities. This programme was incorporated into the labour party manifesto in 1934.

As already mentioned, the Second World War brought to the attention of the authorities the poor state of the nation's health. This was made obvious, as during the First World War, by the large proportion of men who were found to be unfit to join the forces during conscription.

The coalition government, as part of the forward planning for when the war was over, decided that the system of benefits for disabled people needed to be simplified. It was very complex, with benefits being made available by a wide range of different groups. The task was given to Sir William Beveridge, who was a Liberal, a regular broadcaster on the Brains Trust, a journalist and academic. It is said that he had tears in his eyes when asked to take on the work. Not from pleasure, but from frustration that he was not given a more important job in the task of winning the war. It may be this frustration which caused an outpouring of ideas in his report which covered the whole welfare system, from unemployment and disability benefits to pensions, education and the health service. The basic structure of the Welfare State was laid at this time and has altered little since then. Recently, somewhat obscurely, this has been given as a reason for changing it.

The *Beveridge Report* covered the whole of the welfare system.[12] It assumed that the health of the nation was poor, partly because of a lack of access to health services, but also because of the other evils of poverty, unemployment and poor education in a complex knot of interrelated causes. The report was not specific on financing but appears to have assumed that a national insurance-based system would be set up.

The NHS part of the Beveridge proposals was, in many ways, the least radical part of his plan. The social security proposals, especially those relating to unemployment were likely to be the most expensive and the most contentious. Alfred Dolittle in Bernard Shaw's *Pygmalion* best articulated this age-old problem: 'I'm one of the undeserving poor: that's what I am ... I don't need less than a deserving man: I need more. I don't eat less hearty than him; and I drink a lot more.' Governments before and since have struggled with the problem: firstly how to tell the deserving from the undeserving poor and secondly whether they can get away with leaving the undeserving to starve or steal.

▲ 22 How did people respond to the ideas?

The *Beveridge Report*, released on 1 December 1942, included the first outline of a free NHS and was greeted with great enthusiasm. The first 60 000 copies were quickly sold out. The end of 1944 saw 200 000 copies sold. The report described the five giants of want, disease, ignorance, squalor and idleness, and gave specific proposals on how these could be lessened. The whole package of the Welfare State came at a time when the first good news of the Second World War began to come out of North Africa. There was a feeling that the Ministry of Reconstruction would have the opportunity and the blueprint to bring a new hope to society.

▲ 23 How did the hospitals respond to the ideas?

It was envisaged by Beveridge that there would be regional bodies based on medical schools (the most prestigious of the voluntary hospitals) to plan services and develop the health services for a region. The local authority hospitals would stay under the care of local authorities, but the two systems would be co-ordinated by a central Medical Advisory Committee.

At first, the voluntary hospitals rejected the idea of a joint hospital authority, fearing that there would not be true partnership between the public and voluntary hospitals. They assumed that the new regional authorities would come from the local authorities and would favour the public hospitals. It was suggested that the voluntary hospitals should still have to provide some of their own finance. The British Hospitals Association, representing the voluntary hospitals, made the point that it would be difficult for them to attract finances if a free hospital service also existed.

The National Health Service Bill, when it was eventually published in 1946, included the idea that the health service should be free for all at the time when the service was used. The most important policy which the bill brought about for hospitals was to nationalize them and bring them together, in regional groups, covering populations of two to three million, generally with a medical school at the hub. New Regional Hospital Boards were to be set up to administer and plan the development of hospital services.

A second tier of management committees, one for each large or group of smaller hospitals was responsible for the day-to-day operation of the hospitals. The Regional Board appointed these after consultation with the local authority, medical and dental staff of the hospitals concerned. The members of these committees were taken mainly from these groups. The health minister and, under him, the Regional Boards controlled the finances. The teaching hospitals were to have boards of governors, partially appointed as for a Regional Board, with other members nominated by the university. These Boards were to receive the endowments of the hospital concerned to be used as they wished.

Medical schools and teaching hospitals were therefore left to be managed by their trustees. Local government representatives, who, by these changes had lost their own hospitals, were very critical on the grounds that the appointees to the Regional Boards were not democratically elected, although in practice a proportion of the membership of the Boards were drawn from elected councillors. The Royal Colleges welcomed the changes partly because of the high level of remuneration for consultants, who were to be salaried according to the proportion of their time that they gave to the health service. In addition a distinction award scheme was brought in, which was meant to compensate high prestige consultants for the loss of private income which a full-time commitment to the NHS would entail.

▲ 24 How did the GPs respond?

GPs were critical. They were to be paid a small salary and a capitation fee, that is an amount of money for each patient on their lists administered by a Family Practitioner Committee. They lost what few rights they had left to manage patients in the voluntary or local authority hospitals, although they retained their cottage hospitals. The local authorities retained the non-GP community-based services, especially nursing and community medical services, under the direction of the Medical Officer of Health. It was this group that was also responsible for the growing welfare services, later to form social services departments.

This 'tripartite' system of health provision weakened further the contact between GPs and hospital consultants and, in turn, primary and secondary care. There was a belief that doctors who passed their finals and did not want to take any more exams would become GPs. GPs began to feel that they were second class citizens, condemned to the management of diseases that were common, rarely killed patients and were therefore of little consequence.

The white paper for the NHS Act suggested that GPs, who were mainly single-handed, should begin to group together in health centres and hinted that they should be salaried. This was a contentious issue; GPs saw that, if the service was to cover the entire population, there would be little room for private GP practice. It was also thought, at that time, that local authorities would run the GP service locally and that GPs would have no choice about where they would be allowed to practise.

▲ 25 Why was the NHS set up for everyone, not just the poor?

The white paper for the NHS Act stated that everybody 'irrespective of means, age, sex or occupation shall have equal opportunity to benefit from the best and most up-to-date medical and allied services available'. It would be comprehensive, free of charge and would promote good health.

To give the service only to the poor would require testing the means of everyone in the country to see if they could afford it. The use of the means test in the 1930s, when unemployment was very high, was such that no one wished to see its return. As Sir Geoffrey Howe was to say, many years later: 'The principal objection to the means test has always sprung from the fact that it has been so ruthlessly mean.' At that time it was a test of the income of the whole family, so that a few pence earned by any member of the family would reduce the amount received by all. As a result the Welfare State, as envisaged by Beveridge, was equally available to everyone no matter how much they earned. This included the NHS.

It was assumed that the differential between rich and poor would be maintained by the amount put into the service in the form of income tax. Everyone would take out of the NHS what they needed and pay in according to their income. This approach meant that there would be no increased payment for ill people who used the service more. This would have been necessary in a private insurance-based system, where premiums would be highest for those with the worst health. Beveridge originally suggested another option, a compulsory National Insurance system. He believed strongly that people preferred to make contributions to their own benefits. An additional reason was that a married man with two children did not actually pay income tax in the early 1940s until he was earning half of the average wage. In the 1990s the figure is under one-third of the average wage. Beveridge felt that income tax did not cover enough of the population to make it an effective way of compensating the poor. An insurance system also allowed one to 'top up' the basic benefit and receive a little more. Beveridge strongly approved of this approach: that those who saved over and above the bare minimum should be rewarded.

Some people who remember paying directly to Friendly Societies and the Unions when these provided insurance benefits for their contributions claim that that system gave more of a sense of ownership than paying from taxes. You knew who you were paying and what you were entitled to when you needed it. This was lost with the new structure of the NHS which had the appearance that everything was for nothing.

▲ 26 What part did Bevan play?

Aneurin Bevan had been a miner at 13 and at 45 he became Minister of Health in the Attlee government of 1945. The choice of Bevan was a gamble because he was a maverick, 'a squalid nuisance' according to Churchill. He was appointed just as the doctors, through the British Medical Association (BMA), were negotiating on the white paper for setting up the NHS. The doctors were persuaded that an NHS was inevitable but did not like the idea of salaried GPs or of being controlled by local authorities. A great suspicion had built up between doctors and local authorities, partly because of the antagonism between local authority hospitals and the voluntary hospitals and partly because of antagonism to the local authority doctors, the Medical Officers of Health.

Bevan appears to have charmed all around him. He was always well dressed; it is said that he did not possess a pullover. It was he who decided that all of the hospitals had to be brought into state ownership, a proposal not previously put forward by any party or government because of its revolutionary nature. Bevan became a friend with the presidents of the three Royal Colleges, responsible for specialist training. Lord Moran of the College of Physicians was especially influenced and, in turn, influential. The Royal Colleges saw the possibility of spreading the area of influence of specialists far beyond London and the major cities if all the hospitals were to be under the control of a single authority and the specialists were to be well rewarded. They also persuaded him that consultants should be able to do private practice if they wished, in 'pay beds' in the NHS hospitals. He also brought in special 'merit awards' for those specialists who, by taking on full-time work for the NHS, were forgoing their private practice and were doing especially meritorious service.

Bevan thus split the doctors, with the specialists in favour of the NHS, especially since these were not to be under the control of the local authorities. Bevan's main argument at that time was that local authority control would result in too much variation in quality between the different areas: that a series of Regional Hospital Boards run with some autonomy by the Ministry of Health would better ensure equity between the different regions. He was also concerned that local authorities, with their tendency to argue with central government, especially those under the control of the non-government political party, might refuse to implement government policy for the hospitals. Lord Addison, of the eponymous disease, backed him in the Cabinet. Interestingly, the first attempt by local government to run its health service will occur in 1999 in Wales and Scotland when their Assemblies will take over the health service in those areas.

▲ 27 What was the reaction of GPs to the NHS?

Back in 1945, GPs were still not convinced about their part in the NHS. Bevan refused to talk to the BMA until his negotiations with the Royal Colleges were complete. The bill for the NHS Act continued to propose that GPs should receive a basic salary plus a capitation fee, an amount for each patient on their list. A number of GPs suggested that Bevan was acting as Hitler! This reaction was odd in a way, for the proposals were similar to those made some years before by the BMA itself. The GPs did not trust him and strongly believed that Bevan's ultimate aim was to make GPs fully salaried and control where they could practise and the size of their lists. In fact, Bevan appears to have been against this on the grounds that it would mean not giving patients a choice of GP. A capitation fee would mean that good doctors would get more patients and be rewarded for it.

But the BMA was, and is, an organization wide open to impassioned pleas. The Annual Representatives Meeting, the equivalent of a trades union conference, can make policy with a two-thirds majority which is binding on the Association. I have seen impassioned speeches carry the day despite the opinion of the leaders of the Association on the platform. GPs, who probably resented the agreements that their specialist colleagues had obtained, dominated the BMA in those days. In turn GPs who went to the BMA Annual Representatives Meeting tended to be those who were well off and had least to gain and most to lose from the changes. They already had a regular income and feared that they would lose their private patients. Eventually after much argument, which continued until February 1948, 84% of doctors voted in a plebiscite. Of those that voted, 86% were against accepting services under the NHS Act.

Bevan would not budge. Eventually the Royal College presidents, especially Lord Moran of the Physicians, persuaded Bevan to amend the Act so that a whole-time salaried service could not be introduced, except by a new Act of Parliament. The Royal Colleges, for years after, were vilified by the BMA for 'betraying' the GPs. This time a plebiscite showed just over half of the doctors against the Act. The BMA obtained a further agreement, as part of their conditions of service, that GPs' rights to free speech on behalf of their patients would be sacrosanct. Eventually GPs joined in case other doctors should steal their patients. Five weeks before it was due to start, the GPs agreed to take part as independent contractors to the health service.

▲ 28 What differences did the NHS make to patients?

The NHS was the first health system in any western society to offer free medical care to the entire population.

Patients found it hard to believe that they would not have to pay for treatment. My mother had a thyroid operation in a private nursing home in late 1948, despite the existence of the health service. There was also still a belief that the NHS represented a second class service, despite the fact that the voluntary hospitals with their contingent of specialists were all available free.

Other people realized that, at last, they were able to get the spectacles and dental care that they needed. This put quite heavy pressure on the NHS from the start, especially in regard to its costs. Despite this, the queues for free treatment were not as long as some people had feared.

▲ 29 How did the new NHS try to answer the major problems faced by all health services?

There appear to be four main problems faced by any health service (Box 2.1).

Box 2.1 Main problems of health services

- Effects on health other than by the health service.
- Communication, especially between patients and staff.
- Inequality of provision and take up between different groups.
- Rising costs.

The NHS appeared to have the answer to a number of these problems. The Welfare State was a complete package of which the NHS was only part. The idea that housing, education, employment and other social factors affected health was therefore included in the development of the welfare system, which covered all of these areas.

Personal communication and people's understanding of health was not as well addressed by the new health service. The dominant thinking within the professional groups in the NHS was to respond to demands as they arose. Primary care was seen as the poor relation of the specialist service and was split into the GP functions and the district nurses. Both were entirely treatment-orientated. Communication with patients consisted of telling them what they must do in order to treat the problem in question. The district nurses, midwives and health visitors belonged to the local authority. The health visitors were more concerned with some educational and preventative work, but this was confined to helping mothers to look after their babies after the midwife had completed her tasks.

Equity of provision took a stride forward with the setting up of the NHS in two main directions. First, everyone received the service free, so that there was no financial barrier to receiving care. Second, the organization of the service encouraged specialists to move into hospitals away from the larger centres of population, so that highly qualified staff began to spread throughout the country.

Rising costs were problems for the NHS from its inception. The next chapter mentions the results of these concerns, the Guillebaud report and its calming message to the politicians.

3

The 1950s and 1960s: catching up on new developments

▲ 30 What main changes occurred in the NHS in the 1950s and 1960s?

The 1950s and 1960s were a time of consolidation for the NHS. There were some early scares within the first few months of it being set up because of rapidly escalating costs, but these were calmed by the Guillebaud committee, which showed that the increase in spending was generally in line with increases in inflation. The basic management structure remained intact from 1948 until the mid-1970s. This may have been because of the excellence of the structure or because governments then were more wary of interfering with the health service than they are now. The NHS was certainly very popular. It may have been fear of undermining that popularity that kept the politicians from interfering.

Despite this, the big expansions in spending at this time were in education and housing, rather than health. Figure 3.1 shows the amount being spent as a percentage of GDP from 1921 to 1991. There was a general belief, especially among the members of the Labour

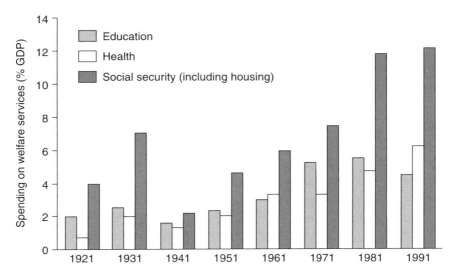

Figure 3.1: Spending on different welfare services, 1921–91.

government just after the war, that good education, good housing and industrial expansion were the priorities. Social security spending and expansion was more rapid than that of the health and education services. This was mainly due to increases in the proportion of elderly people receiving pensions and increases in unemployment pay, both important benefits for maintaining the health of the population. It was not until the late 1960s that a programme of building new hospitals got under way which increased health spending.

▲ 31 What changes occurred in the practice of medicine during this time?

Scientific medicine was finding its feet with a number of effective drugs, especially vaccines and antibiotics further cutting down the rates of infectious disease. These had begun to diminish rapidly after the turn of the century, in response to improvements in the environment. In the past it had been obvious, once the habit of looking objectively at medical practice had begun to develop, that doctors were able to make only slight inroads against diseases which would otherwise run their natural course. Emboldened by changes in disease patterns, which were only partly of their making, they began to see themselves as able to intervene to treat otherwise fatal diseases according to scientific principles. Even at this time, however, Professor Sir Derek Dunlop could claim that the point of a stethoscope was that one should have a 'grey one to go with one's grey suit, a black one to go with one's black suit'. Soon after this, the instrument moved from being a badge of rank to become a scientific instrument.

The general physicians and surgeons, the mainstay of hospital medicine until this time, began to give way to specialists. In the UK, because of the early development and great power of the Royal Colleges, most of the development of new specialties kept the physicians and surgeons separate. Within this structure, the specialties developed according to pathological principles; specialists in diseases of the heart separated from those skilled in diseases of the lungs and from other organ specialists.

Initially, operating on the heart was a very risky business so that the early heart specialists were mainly physicians. Ear, nose and throat specialists, where operating was already well developed were surgeons. This point is interesting because the UK has suffered from such a division in a number of areas. The most recent example of this has been the care of patients with cancer where good medical, surgical, radiological and chemo-therapeutic skills are needed. Because each group has developed from a different base we have been slow to bring units together which can treat the many aspects of the disease. In the past special arrangements have often had to be made for gastro-enterology, where medicine and surgery both make important contributions to the treatment of the same patient over the years.

The 1950s saw the development of a new specialty, geriatrics. This was partly triggered by bringing the local authority long-stay hospitals into the health service and partly by the dedication of a number of very special doctors. These felt that, simply because people were old, they should not be barred from enjoying the benefits of the new effective treatments available in other hospitals. The person most commonly agreed to be the founder of the specialty was a woman, Marjory Warren. The specialty grew slowly at first, gradually overcoming prejudice, until it is now one of the largest specialties in the UK. The UK was the first country to develop such a service. It appears to have been the presence of the NHS which allowed the specialty to develop so effectively nationally.

▲ 32 What brought about the scientific changes in medicine?

The war put an emphasis upon the importance of scientific research for answering practical problems. This was led by men coming out of the forces into higher education and by scientists who came here to escape Nazi Europe which expanded the education and research base in the UK. Figure 3.2 shows how this resulted in a high proportion of

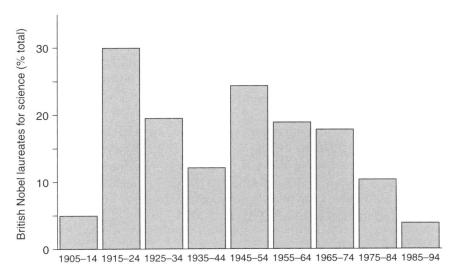

Figure 3.2: Change in percentage of British Nobel laureates over time.

Nobel laureates for the UK in the sciences: medicine and physiology, physics and chemistry. It is of concern that this important factor in the UK has now been considerably reduced.

▲ 33 What non-NHS changes influenced people's health?

In the late 1950s, the consumer boom brought about after the war resulted in high employment and a great improvement in the fitness of the population. Environmental changes were bringing about marked reductions in air pollution. This was rapidly improved by the loss of steam engines and, as new homes started to install electricity and gas, the reduction in coal fires.

The disappearance of pollution was speeded up by legislation for smokeless zones in cities, precipitated, in turn, by heavy smog in London in 1952. The smog contributed to the deaths of several thousand susceptible individuals, especially people with asthma and chronic bronchitis. It led to the passing of the Clean Air Act and of an Alkali Act in the late 1950s. The former sought to reduce the ground level concentrations of air pollution. Pollution from domestic fuel burning was to be prevented by the introduction of smokeless zones in populated areas and industrial pollution was to be prevented by building higher chimneys which would permit dispersal beyond the highly populated areas. The latter, although locally effective, led to effects upon the environment in European countries to the east of the UK, since taller chimneys allowed the prevailing winds to transport sulphur dioxide emissions and deposit them as acid rain. However, smoke concentrations at urban sites in the UK fell by half between 1960 and 1975.

▲ 34 What was happening to general practice?

The 1950s and 1960s were a bad time for GPs.[13] The separation of specialists in the hospitals from the non-specialist GPs occurred at a time when the specialties were beginning to move into exciting, new research work. The GPs felt like, and to some extent were treated as, second class doctors. It was a time when the president of the Royal College of Physicians could describe them as doctors who 'had fallen off the ladder'[14] on their way to becoming specialists. GPs were expected to pay for any additional staff or premises out of a pool, which meant that good practices were penalized. There was little or no development of team work in the practice and no incentive to take on a wider range of approaches, such as preventative work. Training was unstructured and carried out in hospital.

The GPs fought back by forming the Royal College of General Practitioners, which gradually developed an important function overseeing and improving training. It made clear the view that GPs had a body of knowledge of their own which needed to be developed with research and that they required more than just a watered down version of the specialist's training. It was to be some time, however, before membership of the College became a requirement for GPs to practise.

GPs began to leave the profession. Others, in disgust with the BMA, formed a ginger group, the General Practitioners Association; others joined a long-standing rival to the BMA, the Medical Practitioners Union. In the mid-1960s, the GPs negotiated strongly through the BMA, a few for a salaried service, even though they had fought against it 20 years before, some for payment by item of service, but most for a higher capitation fee. They were negotiating with the Minister of Health, Kenneth Robinson who, perhaps luckily, was the son of a GP.

Robinson held out strongly against a fee-for-service payment, despite some pressure from the BMA to do so. This system of payment, where everything that one does is noted and billed separately appears to be responsible for high costs in most of the countries where it is used. It is not difficult to see why. I worked with such a system in Ontario; a secretary was employed full time to follow my every action and note it down. It was easy to inflate the bill, apart from the cost of the secretary. She reminded me never to put two stitches into a cut, for one or two would attract the same payment. I dutifully always put in three. This example was multiplied through my whole practice. This approach was the system of payment that the dentists negotiated in 1948, which caused their costs to rise even more rapidly than the rest of the NHS.

Once the negotiations were complete, the 1966 Family Doctor's Charter allowed 70% of the costs of staff and new buildings to be reimbursed to the GP and higher capitation fees. Stimulated in this way, general practices began to develop. GPs began to employ nurses of their own within the practice. These nurses were initially used for minor tasks within the surgery, such as applying dressings and giving injections, work that had always fallen to nurses. There were a few wild ideas about nurses carrying out assessment visits on behalf of the doctor,[15] but these never really took off. There was a feeling that GPs would not know what to do if the nurses took over some of their routine work.

▲ 35 Why didn't GPs form liaisons with the community staff?

In the 1950s and early 1960s nursing staff, district nurses or health visitors, at that time under the control of the Medical Officer of Health and working for the local authority, were occasionally attached to general practices. Medical Officers of Health felt that such moves would dismantle their empires, and were very resistant to letting their nurses work with the GPs.

There were a number of problems. The nurses were used to working according to strict boundaries, whereas general practice lists contained people from a wide area. Families who had joined the list of a particular GP would, if children left home and moved away, often stay with the same GP, despite having to travel some distance. The local authority nurses might find themselves looking after patients in another area! These problems were really problems of the mind-set of the local authority staff, rather than real ones, but have been used as reasons for not attaching nurses to general practice until quite recently. The majority of district-based staff are now attached to general practice with little or no resolution of the problem; it has simply stopped being a problem.

GPs did not always welcome attached nurses. There was the difficulty of funding reasonable premises for ancillary staff. GPs were quite unaware of what district nurses and health visitors did, or indeed could do. There was professional antagonism between the two groups. This usually took the form of horror stories about what the other side did to 'their' patients.

▲ 36 What was happening to the hospitals under their Regional Boards?

The NHS had inherited a complicated mix of over 2500 hospitals, half of which dated from the 1890s. When Enoch Powell was health minister he ordered a reorganization of the chaotic system of hospitals into a network of large modern units, where the new hospitals were suitable for using the new emerging technologies within medicine. Part of the intention was to reduce the length of stay of patients in hospital, thus reducing costs. Another aim was to reduce the marked differences in care available in different parts of the country. To bring this about, the 1962 Hospital Plan analysed the country region by region to decide on the need for hospitals. The idea of this development was the planning and building of district general hospitals, to this day the centres of hospital care in the UK.

▲ 37 Was there anything in the hospital plan for the GPs?

As well as the district general hospitals, the Hospital Plan[16] suggested the development of large health centres for GPs, sometimes on the same premises as the local authority and later known as community health clinics. This was intended to boost the development of the GP-based primary services. The primary health care teams in these health centres would, it was hoped, develop more preventative services and reduce the pressure on casualty and outpatient departments in district general hospitals.

The enthusiasm for health centres was partially triggered by an enthusiasm for 'polyclinics' developed in the Eastern bloc countries and in parts of Scandinavia, where the great majority of the health care needed by a local population would be carried out, including minor surgery and some specialist outpatient facilities. However, the hospital building programme and more general national financial problems swamped this part of the plan before it could be completed.

▲ 38 Why did prescription charges come in?

The Labour Party made a great fuss about prescription charges when they were brought in by the Tories, in response to continued worries about the cost of the NHS. They did, in fact, abolish them in the mid-1960s, only to bring them back under Kenneth Robinson in the late 1960s. They have remained ever since. It is not clear what they accomplish. There is a very wide range of people exempt from the charges so that only about a third of prescriptions are charged for.

They bring in a small amount of revenue, but there is a feeling that they, in some way, hold down prescription costs. There is some evidence that this may be so, for when charges were scrapped briefly, the cost of prescriptions immediately rose rapidly, only to fall again later when charges were re-introduced. The problem is, of course, that we do not know if the extra prescriptions were for people who needed the medicines or who were simply stocking their bathroom cabinets.

Figure 3.3 shows the proportion of the cost of the NHS covered by prescription charges from the foundation of the NHS. It can be seen that the cost has varied but that it has always been a very small proportion of the total cost of the NHS.

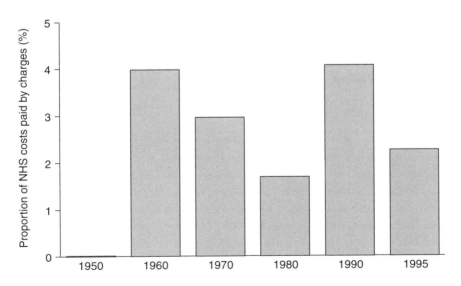

Figure 3.3: Proportion of NHS total cost paid by patient's charges.

▲ 39 How did the NHS at that time deal with the effect of factors other than health care?

It is probably true to say that the main concern of the NHS at this time was to attempt to develop a high quality hospital service, aimed at reducing death and disability. The new specialists, full of enthusiasm, penetrated to the corners of the country determined to bring the most modern approaches to their hospitals. There was a vigorous response by the country to the smogs in the great cities, assisted by new housing and the development of diesel and electric trains in place of steam.

The problems of poverty were being overcome in the middle of the period by rapid economic growth and Harold Macmillan's 'never had it so good' years. This had an important effect upon improving the health of the nation. This boom reversed itself towards the end of the 1960s.

▲ 40 How did the NHS at that time deal with problems of communication?

The growth of the new sub-specialties, based on individual organs – cardiologists for the heart, nephrologists for the kidney, with new intensive care units for the most severely ill – meant that medicine was extremely mechanistic in its approach. The professionals knew best and if one followed their advice one would be well. The belief was that extremely ill people would get better through expert, intensive treatment. Communication was therefore largely one way. The patient listened carefully to what the doctor had to say.

▲ 41 How did the NHS at that time deal with inequity?

Inequity of good hospital and GP care was reducing as high quality specialists and GPs encouraged by the equal pay and conditions in all parts of the country, moved outwards. A few areas were still too unpleasant and poverty stricken to attract good people, but there were not a great number of these. It has already been mentioned that inequities in health, as measured by death and disability, are hardly affected by health services. However, the presence of confident professionals did at least remove some of the fears that people had of ill health. The 1950s saw many people, recently out of uniform, happy to obey the experts. This state of affairs began to change with the advent of 'rock and roll' and the rise of the civil rights campaigns in the USA and elsewhere, pointing out the general inequities of society in the 1960s.

▲ 42 How did the NHS at that time deal with rising costs?

The government was shocked by the early costs of the NHS. Nye Bevan had to revise his first estimate of £170 million a year to £225 million within four months of the creation of the NHS. In 1952, the doctors received a large pay award which alarmed the Treasury. A committee of enquiry was set up under Claude Guillebaud, an economist. His findings showed that the proportion of GDP devoted to the NHS at that time was, in fact, falling. Inflation and extra services had been responsible for the rise in the costs of the service. Indeed, they suggested an increase in capital spending which had fallen well below the pre-NHS equivalent.

This was the first of many panics about spending in the NHS. Guillebaud's report probably saved it when it was still enough of an infant for it to be destroyed. His report also pointed out the tendency for the NHS to meet more of its patients' demands over time. It also scotched the idea that the benefits to the country of a fitter work-force, which would therefore need less care in the future, meant that the NHS would pay for itself.

4

The 1970s: reorganization begins

▲ 43 What main medical changes occurred in the 1970s?

The early part of the 1970s in hospital, just as the latter part of the 1960s, was dominated by the growth of specialist care. This now included units for especially intensive treatment. Examples included coronary care units aimed at preventing sudden death just after a heart attack, renal units for renal dialysis for people with kidney failure and intensive care units for more general problems, especially the care of accident victims. Considerable strides were being made in the development of heart by-pass operations in the surgical field, especially for the treatment of people with abnormal heart valves.

These changes were brought about by the rapid expansion of medical knowledge and the specialization to which this led. The new generation of doctors had trained after the war so that their medical career had not been disrupted, as it had during the previous generation.

These transformations had marked consequences for the training of nurses. The units and the surgical theatre work needed nurses who had considerable technical expertise, which until then had been outside the scope of normal nurse training. Nurses became increasingly skilled by working in the units and attending courses to develop these skills. The large number of extra badges and stripes that they acquired were reminiscent of the boy scouts. In many areas, especially away from teaching centres, nurses had more specialist knowledge than the consultants who were ostensibly in charge.

▲ 44 What main administrative changes occurred in the 1970s?

The 1970s saw the first major administrative change to the NHS since 1948. The government of the day brought in the first of many external management consultants to advise on how better to manage the service. These consultants were given the task of reducing the costs of the NHS and sorting out the complexities of the tripartite system. It was the first of a series of changes to the management structure of the health service, led, it seems, by a belief that any service spending that much money could be organized more cheaply.

The McKinzey report suggested the bringing together of the three health-orientated organizations, with the development of Area Health Authorities as the central focus. These were roughly analogous to counties and their areas contained about half a million people. The Regional Hospital Boards became Regional Health Authorities except in the Celtic countries where the government offices and the Areas split the regional functions. There was talk of introducing an insurance-based system, as there usually is with NHS reorganizations.

The central tenet of the management reorganization was a belief in consensus or team management. Area and Regional Health Teams consisted of the officers of the authority: an administrator, finance director, doctor and nurse. They were expected to reach a consensus on decision-making for the authority. Larger Areas were divided into geographical entities containing about 150 000 people and were known as Districts.

At the same time, Sir George Godber, in a series of Cogwheel reports, outlined a structure for both hospital doctors and GPs to be able to influence decision-making in the Health Authorities. The development of Area Medical Committees and the supporting subcommittees, in theory, allowed every doctor a voice to advise the Authority. These changes were emphasized because of the diminished influence that the profession had on the health authorities as members. The dominance of the hospital doctors over their own administration began to wane as professional administrators, later managers, took over.

These changes in the health service were brought about in 1974. The increasingly specialist nature of the hospital service was beginning, as a spin off, to result in the closure of many of the small cottage hospitals, GP maternity units and long-stay ex-workhouse infirmaries in favour of the large district general hospitals. Some of these were new but many were the original voluntary or local authority hospitals. These district general hospitals now formed the backbone of the Areas and Districts.

The hopes for this new structure were very high at the time. All of the doctors and nurses, with the exception of a tiny number in private practice, were under one authority. The promise of guidance from the medical profession, together with consensus management at the top suggested a recipe for harmony. There was, at the time, a belief that, given the back up of good administration, the senior doctors and nurses could manage the service. Community medicine, derived from a combination of the Medical Officers of Health and the medical hospital administrators in the Regional Hospital Boards, was formed as a specialty, which would help to translate to administrators what it was that doctors wished and vice versa. They would also continue the work carried out by the Medical Officer of Health, assessing the overall health of the population in the Area being served and suggesting means of improving it.

▲ 45 Why was the tripartite system removed?

The late 1960s saw the rapid post-war growth slow down. At the same time the Seebohm report and a Royal Commission on local government suggested the development of the social work profession. This meant the beginning of the end for the empire of the Medical Officer of Health. The social workers developed their own hierarchy, leaving only the school doctors, district nurses and environmental health departments.

The health professionals in the local authorities were increasingly isolated. The image of the public health doctor with its 'rat catcher' and 'drain clearer' image was increasingly unattractive to doctors. The other limb of the tripartite system, the GPs, were also beginning to fight back professionally. It was a time when big organizations were thought to be more efficient. The phrase 'economies of scale' was being bandied about regularly. Interestingly, it seems to be making a comeback in the late 1990s. There was a belief that detailed planning was important. As a result, this reorganization was spelt out in detail with carefully set rules and responsibilities in the Grey Book, which were to be followed rigorously.

▲ 46 How did the medical specialties fit into the new structure?

The development of new specialties, and the spread of well-trained specialists to the country as a whole, required suitable equipment and facilities. The district general hospitals were set up to fulfil these needs. But the hospitals needed to have sensible relationships with the population and community services around them. The reorganization of the NHS in the mid-1970s was intended as an answer to these problems.

With the development of the district general hospitals, the Regional Hospital Boards were seen as too remote and the Hospital Management Committees not professional enough to run these large hospitals. There was a belief at the time that a good administrative structure and planning would bring about greater efficiency.

▲ 47 What changes occurred in general practice?

The reorganization of the NHS brought under one structure the district nurses and health visitors together with the GPs. It was suggested, once again, that as the district nurses and health visitors moved across from the local authorities they should be attached to general practices. The Court Report, in particular, suggested that the care of children should be centred on general practices.[17] This required GPs to take on doctors with a special interest in paediatrics and for health visitors to be directly attached to general practices, to carry out their work with infants and children more effectively. It is a measure of the difficulty of implementing change, which is strongly resisted in the NHS, that these sensible suggestions were once again not implemented. Old health service feuds die hard; the antipathy between the GPs and the doctors and nurses originally working with the local authorities seems to have been fed by successive generations.

In fact, although all doctors and nurses were now in the NHS, the GPs remained separate for all practical purposes under Family Practitioner Committees. They continued to be self-employed contractors with the health service. The main advantage of this, by this time, appeared to be the favourable tax position that self-employed people enjoyed. The 'arm's length' position of general practice over the years must have been, overall, to their disadvantage. They have never been seen as quite part of the NHS.

▲ 48 Did consensus management work?

The promises of consensus management to bring harmony between the professions were not fulfilled. There was quickly a feeling that the advisory structure was too cumbersome. I remember the same policy documents being discussed by similar groups of people in one forum after another. Some of the discontent may have been a feeling engendered by those consultants who had previously successfully exploited the old system and now had to contend with all doctors having the ear of those in charge. It may have been that consensus meant that everyone had a veto. There was some resentment that nurses, who had had little voice until now, had a seat at the top table. Whatever the reason, talk of restructuring began very soon after the system had settled in. Some people say, even today, that it was never given the time to settle in.

Part of the problem must surely have been the rancour between Barbara Castle and the doctors, leading them to strike for the first time in the mid-1970s. There was no real interest in making it work, Mrs Castle because it was a Tory structure, the doctors because they wanted more money.

▲ 49 How did the country at that time answer the problems of health mainly affected by factors other than the NHS?

The main changes during the 1970s were to point out that a number of patients who had been treated for long periods in the NHS did not need to be there, indeed that by their presence their human rights were being violated. This was most obvious for mentally handicapped and mentally ill people but included some elderly people who were kept in long-stay wards without proper care. They were not ill, but were being 'treated' in hospital by medical staff. The first Ely hospital report came out in 1969 and showed the appalling situation in which many patients were being kept.

The pressure to keep these people in the NHS dies hard. Ely hospital still exists as a mental handicap, now called learning disability, hospital and there continue to be occasional concerns about the standard of care there. It is due to close in the next two years, a phrase which haunts those of us who have been around Cardiff for some time.

▲ 50 How did the NHS at that time deal with problems of communication?

In 1971 one of the great communicators of the NHS, Archie Cochrane, wrote a small monograph on the effectiveness of treatment.[18] Archie Cochrane was a medically trained epidemiologist who spent the earlier years of his life working on the problems of lung disease in miners. Later, when directing the Medical Research Council Epidemiology Unit in Cardiff, he widened his interests to other aspects of epidemiology, in particular advocating the use of controlled trials in which the different treatments were randomly allocated to different patients. In this way, he believed, medical care could be concentrated on those treatments where there was objective scientific evidence that they were effective, thus saving the huge amount of time and effort put into treatments which were hallowed by time but which, when tested rigorously, had no effect.

Archie Cochrane was an interesting man. He was one of the well-off, communist sympathizing medics of South Wales. He had a garden scattered with Barbara Hepworth statues and a beautiful collection of paintings. Curiously, after the war he never published a randomized controlled trial, although he helped other people with theirs. He did, however, set up a number of long-term follow-up, so-called cohort, studies in the Rhondda, of which he was rightly proud. In particular he would boast that he had a 100% follow-up of a group of Rhondda women followed up over 35 years. His view was that people should be confident that the treatment that they were getting was effective.

There is a problem here. Even the most effective treatment is not 100% effective. In developed countries, we are mostly trying to treat people with the short-term effects of long-term deterioration. A recent way of describing this has been to talk about the number of people who need to be treated in order to save one life or avoid one major disability. The figures given in this way can be enlightening. Patients who have had a coronary thrombosis, the commonest disease in most Western countries, are given a clot-busting drug, streptokinase, to reduce the size of the damage. This is effective at reducing the death rate according to a large number of randomized controlled trials. However, the number who need to be treated to prevent one patient dying within five weeks of the coronary, is 40. The other 39 get no benefit. It is therefore obvious that, while the treatment is worth giving, on average many people will not benefit from it.

Proof of clinical effectiveness in well-conducted trials is therefore not enough to dispel fear. A proportion, sometimes a high proportion, of patients will not be assisted by the treatment. They will be aware of this, whatever the statistics show for groups of people. Dispelling fear in this situation is not about promising definite cures for everyone. It does not even consist of pretending to all patients that they will definitely be in the minority that improves. Nor, when they do not improve, that it is their fault. All of these approaches are still common in medical care.

The argument is used that patients cannot understand any other approach. This is nonsense. Patients who can understand the treble chance or bet on horses or understand the significance of the sixth ball in the lottery will easily comprehend the idea of the numbers needed to treat.

▲ 51 How did the NHS at that time deal with inequity?

The provision of health care to all, largely free at the point of care, was assumed to look after problems of inequity. The new structure with its Regional, Area and District tiers, with Family Practitioner Committees working under the guidance of each Area was intended to give structure to the NHS. There was someone to run everything at each level, a Regional, Area and District Medical, Nursing, and virtually everything else, Officer. Delegation was the key word and, it was hoped, this would mean that those who knew would do. The universality of the scheme was the key to equality.

In addition, the NHS began to look at how the different parts of the country were funded. Different areas had been, until then, paid the proportion of the pot that they had always had. In the early 1970s, the cost of the health service was £15 per head in the Trent Region and £25 in North East Thames. The new structure allowed the government to try to equalize these differences according to the needs of each Region and, within the Regions, each Area. It attempted to divide the pot by the number of people in each Region, taking into account special groups like elderly people and children and with an additional allowance for areas with high death rates.

▲ 52 What were the priority services?

In the 1970s there was an attempt to divert funds from acute care towards the rehabilitation and long-term care services, which at that time were largely hospital-based, mainly the ex local authority hospitals. This was partially fuelled by the scandals in hospitals for mentally ill, mentally handicapped and elderly people, and partly by the more general attitudes of society to minorities, especially the civil rights movement in the USA and the anti-Vietnam-war groups. They suggested that, given normal social surroundings, many of the problems of these people would be solved. These were, and in some places still are, called the priority services.

These well-meaning moves once again petered out, although a few changes were made, especially the setting up a number of research facilities. These research groups looked at the 'normalisation'[19] of mentally handicapped and mentally ill people, the development of community care, the problems of elderly disabled people and those who care for them.[20] This work laid the foundations for developing the policy on moving mentally handicapped and mentally ill people out of long-term hospital care and, later, the community care part of the NHS and Community Care Act in 1990.

▲ 53 How did the NHS at that time deal with rising costs?

The NHS, during the first half of the 1970s, went through one of its greatest expansions, in relation to GDP. Figure 4.1 shows the changes over time. Curiously, the graph shows that the main proportional increases in the cost of the health service was when the Tories were in power. Over the 48 years shown on the graph, the proportion of GDP given to the health service increased, on average, four times faster per year under the Tories than under Labour. This is an odd conundrum. It may be that the country was more likely to vote the Tories into power when in an expansionist mood, the Labour party when depression loomed.

This finding is quite contentious, as most party political data are, so I include the complete table, for the politicians among my readers to squabble over (Table 4.1).

The Tories showed a 2.19% increase in the percentage of GDP that they gave to the NHS during the 34 years they were in power. Labour showed a 0.2% increase in the 14 years they were in power.

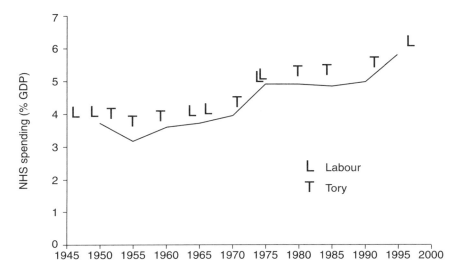

Figure 4.1: NHS expenditure by changes in political party.

Table 4.1: Political party and changes in NHS funding over the first 48 years

Year	Party	Funding (% GDP)	% Change during office
1948	Labour	3.48	0.16
1950	Labour	3.64	–0.2
1951	Tory	3.44	–0.28
1955	Tory	3.16	0.25
1959	Tory	3.41	0.15
1964	Labour	3.56	0.17
1966	Labour	3.73	0.21
1970	Tory	3.94	0.76
1974	Labour	4.7	0
1974	Labour	4.7	–0.14
1979	Tory	4.56	0.55
1983	Tory	5.11	–0.14
1987	Tory	4.97	1.01
1992	Tory	5.98	–0.11
1997	Labour	5.87	–

This is 0.064% per annum for the Tories, 0.014% per annum for Labour, a ratio of 4.5 to 1.

Perhaps the most odd thing about the increase at this time was that the Heath government was making strong noises about cutting public spending. Mrs Thatcher, in probably her most famous move, abolished free school milk for children over eight years of age. The Sun newspaper called her 'the most unpopular woman in Britain', not something it now chooses to remember.

5

The 1980s: how many reorganizations do you want?

▲ 54 What main changes occurred in hospital medicine in the 1980s?

The 1980s were a time when the much vaunted improvements in medical expertise began to look a little hollow. Infectious diseases had been declared beaten, certainly smallpox had been declared eradicated in 1980. Such diseases were assumed to be dead and buried, at least in developed countries. In 1982, the first case of AIDS was detected and the full size of the problem documented by the Centers for Disease Control in the USA. The viruses had fought back at our weakest spot as humans, our unregulated sexuality.

In the UK, a series of other infectious diseases problems followed. Bovine spongiform encephalopathy (BSE) appeared in cattle, and worries about whether it could be transmitted to humans followed close behind. Tuberculosis began to increase again for the first time in years. Diseases that had been around all along received more prominence in the media, especially menigitis and bacteria which were resistant to all antibiotics.

On the positive side there were some early developments using the manipulation of DNA to produce new drugs. The first produced by genetic engineering was human insulin in 1982. Other areas that advanced were in diagnostic imaging, with the development of the magnetic resonance imaging scanner. There was relatively little evidence that these improved the diagnostic process and they were extremely costly but they rapidly spread throughout the country. The ability to take images of complex areas such as the brain, spine and knee joint meant that doctors greatly appreciated the assistance they gave, although in terms of patient well-being evidence suggested that only the images of the head were objectively useful.

▲ 55 What changes occurred in general practice?

It was only in 1980 that GPs were required to go through a period of vocational training in order to become principals in general practice. This required GPs to take on a post-graduate training programme, which was as long and much better organized than most hospital-based specialties. GPs gradually regained their self-respect. There was a gradual increase in the proportion of practices that had nurses working within the practice, although these were still mainly separate from the district nurses and health visitors working in the community services.

About one in five of GPs were working from health centres by this time. However, money for new building was scarce. In its place, GPs were encouraged to borrow money at reasonable rates in the Cost Rent Scheme, to set up their own premises. This they did in large numbers, although the city centre practices were still poorly developed.

In the mean time the government, running out of money once again, brought in a list of medicines which GPs were not allowed to prescribe. Further financial stringencies led to the loss of free eye tests and dental check-ups. There were some suggestions at this time that GPs should be allowed to advertise and set up health care shops with the opticians and dentists under one roof. The GPs began to be suspicious of the government, suspecting moves towards privatization, a change from their suspicion of nationalization in the past.

▲ 56 What main administrative changes occurred in the 1980s?

Money became steadily tighter in the 1980s for the NHS. The management of the health service had, with the 1974 changes, revolved around the idea of consensus management. Mr Roy Griffiths, later Sir Roy, was the son of a colliery worker. He had won an Oxford scholarship and ended up as deputy chairman and managing director of Sainsburys, the supermarket firm. He was asked, in the early 1980s, to look at the management of the NHS in England.[21]

Sir Roy wanted to bring a managerial, businesslike approach to the NHS. He swept aside consensus management as inefficient and slow, in favour of strong management and a feeling that one had to know where, indeed with whom, the buck stopped.[22] General managers were appointed to take over the health service. This meant that, at each level of command, it would be clear who, among the managers at any rate, was in charge.

My memory of that time is that there was much talk of bringing managers in from industry to give the health service the sort of hard-hitting approach said to be common in private companies. This has been said many times in the years that I have been working in the health service. A number of things have blocked it. The first has been that, given an equivalent degree of responsibility, NHS managers get a smaller salary than those in industry. The second is that managers working in industry who do move across find the NHS frustrating in the extreme. Every action the manager takes is scrutinized and often criticized by a succession of people. These may include the next tier of government, the senior doctors, the senior nurses, the Community

Health Council representing the public, a range of voluntary bodies representing other parts of the public and special interest groups. The worst of all is the nearest government department, which, while paying lip service to autonomy and local planning, seems unable to keep its fingers out of the most trivial occurrence, especially if it hits the newspapers. These frustrations occur in industry, but in the NHS all of these groups seem to have more clout with the Secretary of State.

Most of the new people who took over the running of health authorities as general managers were, in fact, the senior administrators who had been working with the consensus until now. The senior managers in the health authorities appointed Unit Managers over the main administrative areas within the health authorities, such as hospitals and community services. This quite minor development was to become vitally important later as these Unit Managers were to become the leaders of what are currently the provider trusts.

The talk, for the first time in the NHS, was beginning to develop around knowing how much things cost and the possibility that efficiency could be improved. Chairmen of health authorities who did not comply found that they were not reappointed. Despite this, some locally elected health authorities held out against changes, especially the tendering out of the hotel, bed and board, services. The process of using local elected people on the health authorities did not last much longer.

▲ 57 What policy lay behind the management changes in the 1980s?

The early 1980s, under Mrs Thatcher, were a time for devolving management. This occurred in schools and the NHS. Some cynics assumed that this approach in a government committed, at least in word, to reducing public spending, meant the devolution of criticism as services were cut back.

Butler has suggested that there were four important developments in the 1980s, under the Thatcher government, that later paved the way for the internal market (Box 5.1).[23] This is not to suggest that these were preparatory moves in a long-term plan. The feeling was of a government flying by the seat of its pants, the political right was wary of too much planning. However, Mrs Thatcher, with her strong feeling for what she believed in, ensured that there were at least some general principles being followed.

Box 5.1 Developments leading to the internal market

- The growing importance of management.
- Income-generating schemes.
- Contracting out services to private companies.

The development of management is mentioned in Chapter 4. The schemes of income generation set up at that time in the UK health service were not very important as means of obtaining cash. They were very important as a way of setting up a new ethos in the health service, of allowing the crossover between the public and private systems to become acceptable.

Contracting out was a more important policy in its own right. In 1983, health authorities were told to use a competitive tendering process to decide who should do their cleaning, catering and laundry.[24] Private contractors competed with the people supplying the existing services. The in-house service usually tendered for the work and often won the right to continue working at lower wages. Some of the trusts made reasonably large financial gains.[25] Despite this, the change was more important as a symbol. Private companies were allowed to invade the NHS. There has been a gradual development of other services being contracted out, although to this day the BMA are totally opposed to contracting out clinical services. It is interesting that the definition of clinical services has gradually tightened over time, so that laboratory services are not now considered clinical.

These changes caused a considerable furore, with Mrs Thatcher constantly being accused of wanting to 'privatise the NHS'. Her answer was to bring in Roy Griffiths, as already mentioned. When he reported back, his main comment was clear. He said that if Florence Nightingale arrived on an NHS ward she would not be able to find out who was in charge. The health service needed managers with power to run the service. For the first time there was to be a line management structure in the NHS instead of a series of lines for each professional group. The theory was that the managers, from whatever background – administration, finance, medicine, nursing or any other – would be managerially in charge of the other professionals. They would not be professionally in charge, however, and therefore unable to interfere in matters of professional judgement. The difference between professional and managerial matters is, of course, impossible to define in many circumstances and effectively means that the senior clinicians are untouchable. Nevertheless, the changes to general management paved the way for the later internal market changes.

▲ 58 Who was Alain Enthoven and why was he important to the NHS?

Alain Enthoven, at present Professor of Public and Private Management at Stanford University, set out his ideas for the future of the NHS in the UK in a monograph in 1985.[26] This was very influential over the changes in 1990. It also helped to reject other changes that were possible candidates, especially, as usual, a possible move to an insurance-based system. He pointed out that the public was very supportive of the NHS. He also said that, as an organization, it was very efficient. Despite this he suggested that it would need to produce even more value for money in the future because he did not believe that such a small cash investment could allow the service to benefit fully from effective new medical technology. It is a common fallacy that health services depend heavily on high technology, whether in the development of machinery or new drugs. The health service as an industry is a low user of technology and many effective new approaches do not require additional technical contributions.[27]

Enthoven also mentioned the difficulties of making changes in the NHS. He gave high praise to the staff and their ability to maintain quality but felt that the structure was too cumbersome for the changes needed to keep up with medical developments. To improve this Enthoven agreed that general managers at authority and hospital levels, which were already being put in place, would help but felt that this did not go far enough. He favoured competitive tendering to put pressure on the service, especially the consultants, to bring about changes. In other words he recognized the need for the managers to have some control over the clinical services. He pressed hard for NHS managers to know their costs and to buy from the private sector where this appeared to be cheaper.

Enthoven also looked at the unequal access to services in the UK. He suggested that people should obtain their services wherever they wished, not only within their own health authority area. He went on to say: 'This line of thinking could lead to an Internal Market Model for the NHS. ... Each District would resemble a nationalised company. It would buy and sell services from and to other health authorities and trade with the private sector.' This was the first mention of an internal market for the NHS. Interestingly he suggested it in the context of competition between different health authorities. Each, he thought, would be vying with each other to persuade patients to travel into their area for the best services. We now know that patients, despite considerable incentives, are very resistant to travelling any distance for their hospital treatment. This contrasts with patients' attitudes to GPs where patients are reluctant to give up a GP they know even if they move some distance away.

Enthoven's idea was that, in competition with others, consultants would impose controls on each other that they would never dream of accepting if the government tried to impose them. He suggested that, in response to competition, clinical freedom would give way to effective control of quality and cost-effectiveness. There is an implication here, as with many people writing about medical costs, that the key to success is to make doctors compete, forcing them to take cheaper options when treating their patients. There is no evidence of them doing this the USA, where they compete more directly with each other for services than in any other developed country.

In his suggestions for reform of the NHS, Enthoven did not envisage two main areas of change that the government introduced. The first of these was self-government for hospitals, developing into trusts. The second was general practice fundholding. These two planks of the reform appeared to evolve as a result of following a logical line of argument within the government. Some people thought, at the time, that they had reached an illogical conclusion.

▲ 59 How did the country answer the problems of health which were mainly affected by factors other than the NHS?

In response to the Alma Ata declaration in 1978 and the call for 'Health for All by the Year 2000', health education and health promotion groups were funded. The health promotion groups were the more radical, calling for the development of community action to ensure that people were aware of health issues – from the things that governments did, down to their own lifestyles. They hijacked a great deal of variable evidence on, for example, the prevention of heart disease by dietary means. There was a tendency for them to make claims for the prevention of disease by simple changes in lifestyle, such as jogging and eating, which could not be sustained by any real evidence. There was also a tendency in the movement to connect health with fitness, goodness and sexiness. There was just a suggestion that ill people might have themselves to blame. In this way they were similar to the present day 'environmental' movement: a mix of puritan prejudice and a grain of truth.

The AIDS epidemic, with its requirement for the personal prevention of disease by safe sex fitted in well with the movement and was partly responsible for its ability to attract funding. Eventually, towards the end of the 1980s the movement began to peter out. It was a pity it was done the way it was. Some of the messages, especially that people can more fully understand their own health, were valuable and have been largely lost. The demise of the high profile groups was largely a result of their tendency to use government money to attack government policy, for instance on tobacco or sex education. This was not a popular approach with Mrs Thatcher's government.

At about this time, the BMA, which had an increasingly bad image for being interested only in money, made a determined effort to change. It began to develop its health policy arm with reports about issues connected with, but not in, the health service. There were reports on boxing, seat belts, drink-driving, banning tobacco advertising and the medical effects of nuclear war. The BMA showed a parallel interest in the topics that the health promotion people were advocating. These valuable reports began to give the BMA a more radical image and to bring it into conflict with the Thatcher government. The BMA was now strongly supportive of the NHS, both in fact and as policy. It became and remains a central belief of the BMA that what is good for the NHS is good for doctors and vice versa. It is, of course, in the interest of the BMA for the public to see it this way too.

▲ 60 How did the NHS deal with problems of communication?

Ian Kennedy, in his Reith lecture in 1980, suggested that there should be a new relationship between doctors and patients. Patients, he said, should take more responsibility for their own lives and should challenge the power that doctors held.[28] As is usual with Reith lectures, the content was not new, it was the fact that it was given as part of an 'establishment' talk that was important. Many other people over the years had knocked the medical establishment and their inability to deal with patients, except on a mechanistic basis. The greatest exponent of this approach was Ivan Illich in the 1970s who believed that doctors did more harm than good.[29] Just after this, from within medicine Thomas McKeown cast doubt on the claims of doctors to have had an important impact upon mortality or morbidity.[30]

The moves to devolve the control of the health service to smaller units under managers did not make it any easier for patients or the public to question the decision makers in the NHS. The people in charge of treatment, the specialists and GPs, were still in complete control over the care of their patients. The patients, in reality, had little control about which doctor they went to see, or which consultant they were referred to.

There was, and still is, ample evidence for the inability of doctors to communicate with patients. A study carried out in the late 1980s showed that about a third of people going into hospital wanted more information than they were given and about a third of those received no adequate explanation.[31] There is a problem. Although ignorance certainly increases fear and there is ample evidence to prove that doctors have feet of clay, we need to build another approach which depends more on mutual respect and understanding. Saying that doctors are all rubbish will not relieve the resulting fear that patients will have. The NHS needs to give part of its organization to translating the complex issues of health care so that people in general can understand. Interestingly, as the health promotion movement showed, this rapidly gets one involved in the political arena and, if funded by the government, rapidly closed down. It is likely that such an organization can only come from the independent sector, either an academic or private organization.

▲ 61 Why do doctors never explain what is going on?

The relationship between doctors and their patients is complicated. The view of doctors – seriously held in the 1940s by the TV doctor, Dr Kildare – that a surgeon had 'Life in one hand and death in the other' vanishes slowly in the UK, especially among older people who make up the majority of patients. Generally, patients have less difficulty talking to and understanding GPs than consultants in hospital. Part of the reason for this is that the doctors in hospital do not know the patients they meet and therefore find it difficult to talk in simple terms to them. As already mentioned, most doctors belong to a different social group from their patients. Their values and interests are quite different, from the type of food that they eat, the sort of sport that they enjoy to the television programmes they watch.

With that sort of background it is no wonder patients do not understand what a doctor says to them. Most patients are frightened, terrified of being told some things: that they are going to die, that they will endure pain. There is not much time. The NHS usually ensures that patients have ten minutes at most to talk to a doctor, most often less.

▲ 62 Are we choosing the right doctors?

We may be choosing the wrong people to be doctors. Medical schools in the UK, in contrast with the situation in the USA, have no difficulty recruiting students. The competition depends upon good examination grades, so that the students who enter medical schools are chosen from those who are best at chemistry, with the addition, most commonly, of biology, physics or maths. These subjects are not likely to help students to develop their communication skills, nor are those most naturally adept at communication likely to choose them.

In the UK, training for a GP lasts at least eight years before he or she becomes a principal. For a consultant, the time will be more. During their training, doctors learn a great number of technical and scientific facts but, although recent changes have put more emphasis upon communication skills as a separate package in the curriculum, the central core of the course is about learning facts and applying them.

Another problem with communication is that patients often assume that the doctors know the answers to the questions they most want to ask. In hospital it is usually the middle range of doctors, the registrars, who know most about what is wrong with their patients. The specialists are not as immediately available, partly because they have outpatients or operating theatre work to do, partly because they may have teaching and other commitments away from their home hospital. The most junior doctors often have to cover a number of other firms at night so that they find it very difficult to keep up with their own patients. In hospital wards the turnover is so rapid that even the nurses may have little time or useful information to impart.

▲ 63 How did the NHS deal with inequity in the 1980s?

In 1980, a report set up by the previous Labour government and chaired by Sir Douglas Black was published on inequalities in health.[32] I remember asking several times for a copy of a poorly bound, typewritten report in a lurid purple colour. I ordered four more and sent them to colleagues who were having difficulty getting them, feeling very self-congratulatory that I was spreading data which the government wanted suppressed. The new Thatcher government was not interested in finding unmet needs shortly after getting into power. The response by the government to the report was that it pointed out in considerable detail the problems that poverty caused in relation to health, but did not say why there was a connection, therefore nothing could be done. The report was published again two years later as a paperback.

It is perhaps a sign of improvement in this area that the Government Statistical Service themselves published a follow-up book on health inequalities in 1998.[33] This is an excellent book but shows that, if anything, the health inequalities between the rich and poor in the UK have increased since 1948, indeed since the early 1980s.

▲ 64 How did the NHS at that time deal with rising costs?

The middle and late 1980s were a time of considerable crisis for the NHS. A succession of Health Ministers continued to tighten up the money available. Mrs Thatcher was reluctant to make changes to the NHS, because of its popularity, yet was eventually forced to set up a committee of ministers to look into possible ways of getting around the problem of keeping the NHS going without increasing public spending. There were temptations to increase the private sector in some way or to go for an insurance-based, rather than a tax-based, system. Both would have a major impact on patient's awareness of the changes. The ideas that became gradually accepted had the benefit of being invisible to the way that patients would pay for or obtain their care.

I have mentioned that Alain Enthoven had suggested the idea of an internal market within the health service in the early 1980s. Purchasers who have the money and providers who compete for that money were common currency in education, where schools acted as the providers. The idea of making hospitals independent providers is said to have come from a surgeon, Ian McColl from Guys Hospital, previously well-known in medical circles as a strong advocate of medical audit, where doctors assess each other's work in a structured way.

In July 1988, Kenneth Clarke became Secretary of State for Health. He was completely against increasing privatization, mainly because allowing people to opt out of NHS care would take out the mainly fit, wealthy contributors leaving the unfit and poor to be looked after by the NHS. This is a quandary for all countries running a health service. A two-tier service is not just unfair, it also makes the lower tier very expensive, while giving a poorer quality service than the upper tier. The NHS appears to manage this better than most. Kenneth Clarke is credited with thinking up the idea of GP fundholders, although Alan Maynard and Nick Bosanquet, both health economists, had mentioned it previously at a conference in 1984.

The launch of the ideas leading to the new reorganization, in January 1989, was given huge publicity but, in contrast to the 1974 reorganization, there was little detail. The next few years saw policy being developed as it went along. But what of the rising costs of the health service? The reorganization did not provide more money but the crisis disappeared. Perhaps the answer to needing more money in the health service is simply to think of something else to catch people's attention.

6

The 1990s: the market will provide, then stopped providing

▲ 65 What was the internal market?

The health authorities, until 1990, oversaw the planning of the health service and delivered the services. Within each authority were a varying number of units: hospitals, community services, ambulance services. The purchaser–provider split set up an internal market by separating the central planning and financing functions of the health authority from its health services provision. The centrally based group were the purchasers, the units were the providers. Initially the term 'procurers' was used for the new health authorities. Thankfully, for those of us who had to tell people what we did for a living, this term rapidly disappeared.

▲ 66 Who were the purchasers and providers in the internal market?

The task of the purchasers was to reach the best compromise between cheapness and quality for each of the services they bought. The providers – hospitals, community units and others – split off to form self-governing trusts. These trusts competed with each other, as part of the internal market, for the money held by the health authorities. The health authorities decided which of the competing providers should get the money by setting up contracts, which the providers could, in theory, compete for. The home purchaser paid for people who belonged to one area but were taken ill in another.

These changes were set up under the NHS and Community Care Act 1990. At health authority level, the Act made changes to the boards of health authorities. Before the Act, boards of 15 to 20 members ran the health authorities, many with a special political or professional interest in the NHS. Some were local councillors. They were often slow to reach a consensus, because of their conflicting political ideologies. Executive and non-executive board members replaced these. The executives were and still are the full-time managers at the top of the organization, headed by a chief executive. They usually include a finance director, a medical director, a nursing director and one other, often someone involved with the development of the trust or marketing. They are balanced by the non-executive directors, who are part-time, in theory giving about a half day a week to the work.

▲ 67 What precipitated those changes?

The great pressure put on Mrs Thatcher to provide more money for the NHS in the late 1980s has already been mentioned. In some ways the changes were much more radical than people had expected, but they did leave the NHS intact. The possible major change of a move away from taxation funding to an insurance base, which might have been expected from Mrs Thatcher, did not happen. Some of the reasons why this may have been so have already been mentioned. In addition, some have commented that, when it came to making changes which the public valued, Mrs Thatcher was quite conservative.

▲ 68 Who was in charge of the health authorities and trusts?

Elected representatives have never run the health service in the UK. Until the changes ushered in by the NHS and Community Care Act 1990, the people who ran the health services locally were taken from three main constituencies: the local authorities, local eminent doctors or other professionals and a mixture of the great and good, including prominent trade unionists. Often only the chief officer of the health authority attended board meetings.

The problem was that the authority members would often represent a party or professional interest, rather than the interests of the health of the local patients or the smooth running of the local services. The members sometimes appeared to be in a state of siege with their officers, with the officers attempting to hide the real consequences of actions inside complex technical language. Some members of authorities held pre-meetings, one for Labour members and the other for Conservative members, to decide upon which way to vote, similar to that of more political forums, such as parliament or local authorities.

▲ 69 How were the new chairmen and directors chosen after 1990?

With the advent of the NHS and Community Care Act 1990, the Secretary of State chose and still chooses the new chairmen of both health authorities and trusts. There are usually five executives and five non-executives on each board with the chairman holding the balance. The executive directors are the people who oversee their part of the service, a chief executive in charge with a finance director, director of medicine, director of nursing and another director who looks after administration or the development of the organization.

The non-executive directors, after the 1990 Act, were generally chosen for their business expertise. Some had previously been involved in the old health authorities. The theory was that the new authorities and trusts would be run much more along the lines of businesses, rather than as the traditional model of public service providers. The requirements of the internal market meant that financial and managerial expertise, in particular, were prized. Most non-executive members of authorities and trusts therefore came from that sort of background and tended to favour the Conservative party.

It would be naive to suggest that the government were not aware of the advantages to them of using a group for non-executive members who were likely to be its supporters. There has always been a strong tendency in the UK for the government of the day to use its patronage to ensure that its own supporters are put into positions of influence. The unusual thing about the UK in this regard is that the government usually denies it vehemently. The Labour government, when it came to power in 1997, rapidly got into arguments because people accused them of appointing only Labour supporters to vacant non-executive posts.

The idea of the development of trusts was that patients would be seen as customers who could take their custom elsewhere and must therefore leave reasonably satisfied with the care they received. However, patients still had little direct control over the care they obtained. The theory was that their GPs, especially those in fund-holding practices, would be likely to take notice if a patient was unsatisfied with his or her treatment, when the system ensured that the GP could use another trust as part of the internal market.

▲ 70 Where did the 'market' fit in?

The buyers and sellers in the NHS market were not as free as those selling their wares in Petticoat Lane. Indeed, one might think that it is a strange market where all the goods are free over the counter and everyone, whether buying or not, helps to pay for the goods on the 'never never', as taxes. The good news for those paying is that the total amount of goods paid for each year is restricted to a maximum sum at the beginning of the year. As a result the sellers will, on occasion, run out of things to sell. In that situation, buyers have to queue until more goods arrive. I will resist the temptation to squeeze this analogy into whether the goods are cheap and shoddy or of good quality. Nor indeed whether they would be legal under the Sale of Goods Act as 'fit for their purpose'.

The arrangements for NHS trusts were set up, especially in their system of capital funding, so that they did not have a natural advantage over other providers outside the health service.[34] However, the NHS trusts are several orders of magnitude bigger than the private and voluntary providers and in most cases can provide a cheaper and more comprehensive service than the independent groups.

▲ 71 What changes occurred in hospital medicine during this time?

An important movement within all of medicine, but which had most impact on hospital medicine arose at this time. This was a concentrated effort to follow the ideas that Archie Cochrane had put forward in the 1960s and early 1970s on the objective measurement of the effect of medical care. Looking after patients according to the best clinical effectiveness is defined in Box 6.1.

Box 6.1 Definition of clinical effectiveness

The conscientious, explicit and judicious use of current best evidence in making decisions about the care of individual patients. Practising it means integrating individual clinical expertise with the best available external evidence from systematic research.

Source: Sackett D, Richardson W, Rosenberg W *et al.* (1997) *Evidence-based medicine: how to practise and teach EBM.* Churchill-Livingstone, New York.

In other words, you have to know your science first and apply it to patients, bearing in mind their unique differences from the average, which the science is based on. The reasons for the recent increase in interest in trying to improve the scientific basis of the routine treatment that we give revolves around a number of changes in health care that have been increasing over a number of years, but which are increasingly impossible to ignore. These are summarized in Box 6.2.

I have previously mentioned that there is a problem with reliance upon scientific clinical trials for treatment when one applies it to oneself as a patient. With modern forms of treatment the advantages of different drugs are often not very great, although they are better than doing nothing. An extremely effective treatment will often only improve one person in five on average. Some people describe the effectiveness of care as the 'number needed to treat' (NNT); an improvement of one in five has an NNT of 5. The problem for an individual patient is, of course, that four of the patients receive no benefit. For an individual, a chance of one in five is quite small.

Box 6.2 Increased interest in clinical effectiveness

- A large international group of committed people with an interest in the subject.
- Increasing concerns about the costs of health care, especially from the USA, where publicly funded health care appears to be out of control: the lower tier problem mentioned above. A suggested answer is to restrict what the public bodies will fund to those things which are of 'proven effectiveness' in the assumption that this will be less than is provided at present.
- A rapid and costly rise in complaints and legal suits, especially in the USA. This has led to a search for an agreed 'right' way to give the different forms of health care so that doctors are legally safe. One response to this has been the rapid development of guidelines of good practice, akin to the Highway Code for drivers.
- Evidence of dramatic variations in the number of medical interventions performed in different places for the same problem. Table 6.1 shows the great variation in the time people spent in hospital for classes of disease in four developed countries. There is no good evidence of the right length of stay but such huge average differences suggest something is wrong.
- A huge rise in scientific data about health care; over a million articles a year in medical journals alone, making it difficult for medical staff to keep up with the latest changes. Those working in the subject therefore assess which are the important findings using scientific criteria.
- The public now has more knowledge of health care. This trend was again led by the USA but the availability of the Internet and an increase in medical articles in the media means that doctors and nurses have to struggle to keep their knowledge ahead of their patient's.
- Best practice diffuses slowly through the medical profession so that, as change accelerates, it has become important to help the staff keep up with postgraduate training.

Table 6.1 Variations in length of stay in hospital for certain conditions in different countries

	Length of stay (days)			
	UK	USA	Canada	Japan
Neoplasms	12.2	10.5	16.2	51.7
Mental disorders	50.3	11.6	24.7	333.3
Infections and parasitic diseases	9.6	6.9	10.5	117.6
Diseases of the blood	12.6	7.2	11.1	41.7

▲ 72 What changes occurred in general practice: why fundholding?

The American management gurus did not seem willing to suggest changes to primary care, especially the GP service. The UK service has always been unusual in that the great majority of people going into hospital, the expensive part of the service, have to be seen by GPs first. It is believed that this set-up has been partly responsible for keeping down prices in the NHS. Nevertheless, an important part of the NHS and Community Care Act 1990 was the development of GP purchasing. This allowed GPs to apply for what was known as fundholding status if they had a list size of at least 5000 patients. This number was gradually reduced as the fundholding approach grew. A later addition was that GP practices with as few as 3000 patients could opt to hold the budget for outpatient and community care only.

Fundholding practices were allowed to act as purchasers of secondary services. They were given a budget taken from the health authority allocation. This was, initially, to cover the cost of certain non-emergency inpatient and outpatient care. It also covered the cost of their prescribed drugs and the staffing costs of the practice. They drew up contracts with the hospital or community trusts specifying the cost of the service and its quality. At the present time (1998), with the fundholding system abolished, GP fundholders purchase about 8% of the trusts' budgets. Just over half of the population are registered with fundholding practices.

▲ 73 How did the Labour government change things in 1997?

The Labour government, which came to power in 1997, took steps to abolish the internal market, but has kept the split between purchasers and providers. It abolished GP fundholding. In 1998 it published separate White Papers for England, Wales, Scotland and Northern Ireland on their policy for the NHS. The main points of the White Papers were similar, although there were detailed differences. Purchasing is to be carried out by GP purchasing groups covering populations of about 100 000. The purchasing groups, called Primary Care Groups in England, were to include representatives from a wide range of people involved in primary care: GPs, community nurses, pharmacists and many others.

In England, these groups were divided into four main types: those who were to give advice to health authorities on what to purchase, those who would purchase directly some services; those who would purchase the majority of services for the health authority in their area; and those known as Primary Care Trusts. The last group is new and it is not yet clear exactly what their function will be. A small, but important, part of the White Paper was a suggestion that GPs will be cash-limited in future. In other words, each general practice would have a budget to which they must keep. This was a new change for general practice; except for GP fundholders, the budget for general practice has always been open-ended.

This aspect of the White Paper may prove to be the most controversial because some GPs will miss the freedom of being fundholders, especially as this will involve disbanding the team that they collected together to make fundholding work. They are also beginning to resent being told to join commissioning groups. Under the previous system becoming fundholding was, in theory, voluntary. The new commissioning groups, if they are to work, will require most GPs to be involved in purchasing. It seems likely that a proportion of GPs will have no interest in this sort of work and will not see it as their job. The commissioning groups will largely be taking over the functions of the health authorities. Presumably it is the intention of the government that the commissioning groups will increasingly do all of the purchasing and that the health authorities' power will wane. This means that the commissioning groups will need finance experts and experts in assessing health needs, the public health doctors, as well as the many groups of primary care workers. I can understand some GPs being keen to spend time in long, boring meetings when commissioning services for their own fundholding group. I find it unlikely that many will relish the same meetings for an area containing 100 000 people, especially if the health authority still has most of the power.

It has been suggested that consultants from the local trust will also need to have a voice, although the government has resisted this. Local authorities will need to be involved, as most of the commissioning groups will be coterminous with the local authority area. The potential for in-fighting appears to be immense.

▲ 74 What were the strengths of the internal market?

The main strength of the internal market was that it was reasonably easy to understand. The strength of the internal market for purchasers was that they could specify what they bought in as much or as little detail as they wished. The purchaser had, theoretically, a free rein. There were limits built into the system, including giving any provider six months warning about major changes proposed in the service. The Department of Health also issued general strictures not to undermine the viability of trusts and in practice purchasers have, if anything, been gentle in their demands on providers. After all, only a few years back they were colleagues in the same organization. Many people, especially in management, moved from one side of the service to the other. GP fundholders have not been as moderate, but they had the benefit of knowing that they represented only a small part of a trust's budget.

All areas and providers have their black spots. These black spots may be a specialty, a service or an individual. The internal market did not solve all of the problems, but it did allow the purchasers to put pressure on a provider if a poor service was consistently provided. They could remove the contract from one provider and give it to another. In addition, providers were required to develop and try to sell new ideas.

My own view is that there was one particular aspect of the internal market which was a success. The large monolithic health authorities were split up into smaller groups, usually based on a hospital or the community services in an area. These usually made more sense to the people working for them than the larger units. The competition between trusts also lent coherence to the people working in that trust; they knew where their organization began and ended. Most of the trusts were small enough to be managed efficiently. There is a 'lumping' move afoot at the moment, which will lose these advantages. I disagree with Nye Bevan's adage that I would 'rather be kept alive in the efficient if cold altruism of a large hospital than expire in a gush of warm sympathy in a small one', but he was speaking before the age of antibiotic-resistant bacteria.

▲ 75 What were the weaknesses of the internal market?

In practice, some aspects of the internal market were disappointing. Some trusts had been fast to develop new, exciting approaches to the delivery of services, but they were a minority. Generally the trusts have been defensive, worrying about their budgets and trying to keep their heads down. Some people have suggested that the required changes in the culture of the NHS would have taken longer than the experiment allowed. Even during the development of the internal market, changes were being made to the composition of health authorities so that it was easy for a trust that was resistant to change to prevaricate until it was too late to agree major changes to the annual contract.

The built-in competition between providers also made collaboration between them difficult. Having said this, collaboration between two hospitals or other parts of the service before the internal market was not very good. Each unit within the NHS contains a large number of professionals who, either from pride or fear of competition, is often defensive of the way their own establishment does things and is resistant to change. This remains, market or no market.

The internal market caused problems for GP fundholders. They had to make overt choices when purchasing one of two alternatives. This is a disadvantage for the losing trust if the choice is not explained to the public promptly and clearly. Trusts that lost services that they had provided for some years tended to cry foul to the press. Sometimes the decision not to give a service to a particular trust, even at the individual patient level, hit the headlines. This is only a weakness of the service if the purchaser or provider in question is unable to give coherent reasons for their decisions. Unfortunately, there is no tradition within the health service for doing this, so that patients often had a distorted view of what was going on in the service.

The internal market also required an overt emphasis on costing. Health authorities, trusts and GP fundholders produced annual reports, which had to include detailed costs. This was new for the NHS with a long tradition of 'getting it roughly right then adjusting it later'. This emphasis upon money appeared to make the service appear less altruistic than it had been in the past. There has been a long tradition in medicine, from the days of the voluntary hospitals, of giving free treatment and the NHS inherited much of this convention.[35]

Mrs Thatcher's favourite image of the market was of a group of costermongers vying with each other about the price and quality of their goods to sell their wares. In this model, price is not something one mentions as an afterthought, it is shouted as part of the marketing. Despite this, the internal market in the NHS was different from such a free approach. It had to keep within budget and to provide a full range of medical care free at the point of use. It is hard to envisage a group of costermongers developing a managed market under such constraints. It might just do so under heavy threat from the local spivs. It is interesting to surmise about who has that rôle in the health service.

▲ 76 Why do governments reorganize the NHS so much?

The tendency of the NHS, despite various forms of reorganization, is always back towards the monolithic. All big organizations with a hierarchical structure seem to go through cycles of splitting and lumping in turn. The NHS has always been very closely ruled by the government of the day. Generally the Conservatives have tended to be splitters, while the Labour party have been lumpers, although there are exceptions.

An exception is in the provision of different types of service by the local authorities in different counties. Figure 6.1 shows the relationship between the proportion of Labour councillors in a county and the number of home helps provided in that area. It should be said that, for the sake of political balance, the number of residential home places was closely allied to the proportion of Tory councillors. The data on residential homes are no longer possible to collect as most nursing and residential homes have now been moved out of the local authority control to the independent sector.

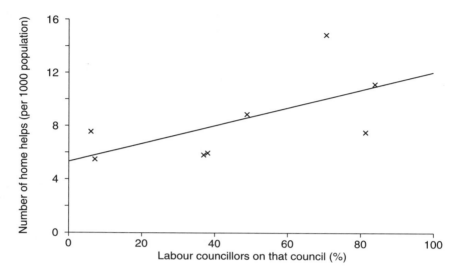

Figure 6.1: Relationship between proportion of Labour councillors and home helps in a Welsh county.

▲ 77 How did the country answer the problems of health mainly affected by factors other than the NHS?

The health promotion and health education movement, from being fêted when they first began to develop their work, now found themselves at loggerheads with the government on a series of issues. A number of the leaders of the movement resigned under clouds of varying blackness due to trying to promote issues with the public which ran counter to government policy or what the government perceived as the public taste. An example of this clash was the release of booklets giving advice on sex matters to youngsters in schools. This was aimed to be simple and clear, the very opposite of the British approach over centuries. The booklet was withdrawn.

The later years of the 1990s have seen a resurgence of interest in health inequalities, which is mentioned in more detail below.

▲ 78 How does the NHS deal with problems of communication?

Personal communication between patients and doctors does not seem to have improved over the period of the NHS. The General Medical Council (GMC), which oversees the training of doctors, came to recognize that it is a problem in the 1990s. A report to overcome these problems recommended considerable changes in the way that medicine is taught in medical schools in the UK.[36] The report made the point that the main focus of medical education up to now has been understanding disease processes as they affect individuals, diagnosis and management. It stressed the reawakening of the wider interest of 19th century doctors in the health of populations and the epidemic, social and environmental hazards that affect them. It said that public health should be reinstated as a priority subject in the planning of medical services.

The report pointed out that in future there are likely to be more overlapping skills and responsibilities. It also emphasized the importance of teamwork between professionals and the priority to be given in future to learning to train aides and relatives, who may have little or no training except for carrying out specific tasks for a single relative. This type of approach will be important so that expensive professional skills can be used to their best advantage.

The GMC report also stated that there has been a drive within medical education towards an unrealistic degree of completeness so that medical graduates, on the day they graduate, are trained in every specialty that they may later wish to enter. It suggested that, as all specialties now require higher training, most of the factual learning previously in the undergraduate course can be brought in at a later stage. It pointed out that the knowledge base of medicine changes quite profoundly over quite short periods of time, so that the ability to relearn and adapt is more important than absorbing today's facts. It emphasized a required 'core' of learning and closer integration of the scientific part of the undergraduate curriculum and that part which has always been traditionally taught as an apprenticeship system. In particular, it pointed out the central importance for doctors of communication with patients.

Another change is the emphasis upon project work and the requirement for students to study in some depth a small number of aspects of the work that they do. This would not be the same for all students, indeed diversity in the approaches that different students take is to be encouraged. Another principle is towards self-directed learning.

Other parts of the GMC recommendations suggest the crossing of traditional departmental boundaries, with interdisciplinary collaboration in planning courses to break down the barriers between traditional specialties or, at least, lead to new alliances between different groups. There are particular suggestions that medical students should be brought into contact with families in the community in which, for instance, a baby is expected or which contain an elderly or disabled member. They make the point that skills are essential to the needs of good medical practice and also suggest the development of two new important areas of work: the idea of man in society and the importance of public health. They suggest that there should be much more emphasis upon the importance of the prevention of disability and minimizing handicap during the rehabilitation process.

▲ 79 How does the NHS deal with inequity?

The mid-1990s saw an increased interest in the inequities of health between different groups of people, accelerated by the publication of a book by the Government Statistical Service on inequalities in health.[33]

It is a step forward that a government department, in contrast with the Black Report, which was initially suppressed by the government, should publish data on the subject.

This report shows that health, in terms of mortality, has been improving steadily for a number of years for all groups, but that the improvement has been faster in well-off people compared with poor people. The difference between them has therefore widened. Figure 6.2 shows the increasing difference between social classes I and II and social classes IV and V for men in terms of life expectancy. The difference for the period 1972–5 was 3.9 years whereas for 1987–91 it was 5.2 years.

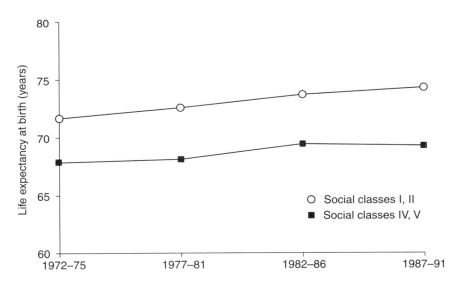

Figure 6.2: Life expectancy for different social classes: males.

▲ 80 How does the NHS deal with rising costs?

Costs continue to rise in the NHS. At the present time there has been a slight acceleration upwards in the cost of the NHS (Figure 6.3) if a comparison is made with 1949 prices. Figure 4.1 showed that spending in the 1990s has increased in relation to GDP.

The Tory spending plans, after the 1997 election, were to cut back on spending in the NHS, once in power. When Labour won the election and formed a government they decided to keep to the low rates set by the Tories. The rapid rises in costs also suggest that either the internal market did not force costs to stay down or else that the system, with its large number of checks and balances, had not really settled in. Some observers have suggested that costs will not be greatly altered until managers are allowed to take charge of treatment costs,

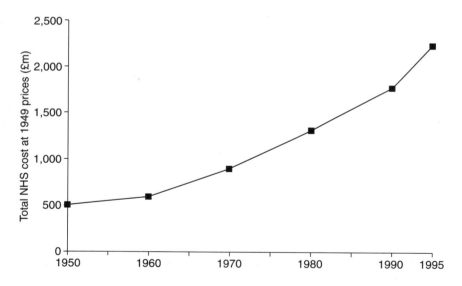

Figure 6.3: NHS costs at 1949 prices.

but this will be a hard-fought battle with no likelihood that the managers will win.

It has already been mentioned that the majority of these costs are for paying nurses. The internal market did try to hold down staff costs by bringing in local pay bargaining and restricting pay rises to nurses. The political fuss caused by these attempts meant that local managers were regularly told by central government what their local bargaining should consist of. This became more and more ridiculous year by year. The Labour government has now reinstituted central bargaining, so that little more can be gained in increased efficiency from competition for efficiency between different parts of the NHS.

7

The 2000s

▲ 81 What changes are patients likely to see in the 2000s?

There is no doubt that patients will be better informed about health matters and better able to get highly expert advice about their health without having to go to their GP or anyone else giving primary care. The data revolution, especially the Internet, is the main reason for this. The GPs and junior hospital doctors that I teach already describe patients coming to them with inch-thick piles of paper which describe their symptoms and several possible methods of treating those symptoms. A local newspaper recently quoted a woman with multiple sclerosis being very rude about a hospital doctor who had told her that dietary modification does not help people with the disease. She disagreed with the doctor, stating that two experts on the Internet had 'proved conclusively' that diet had a place and that she was going to follow the advice of these experts.

A doctor will have to be prepared, in future, to describe the constant battle within medicine to check potentially harmful and useless treatments: the constant battle against quackery and enthusiasts hoping to make their reputation or fortune with the latest gimmick. And a wise doctor will spend some time explaining the subtler problem of potentially useful treatments that only work for a small proportion of people. The problem with this approach is that the most expensive part of the health service is the professionals' time and such explanations will take a lot of it.

▲ 82 What changes in science are likely?

Changes that are already well advanced can be extrapolated to the future. The first of these suggests less invasive interventions in the future. Surgery is moving from keyhole to micro to external. Lasers, which can destroy tissue internally without cutting the skin, are developing rapidly. Flexible narrow catheters in blood vessels and the gut are able to get to increasingly inaccessible parts of the body without major trauma, often without cutting the skin.

The replacement of diseased organs will obviously continue. The possibilities of growing these tissues from animal or human fetal tissue with genetic modifications to prevent rejection are being debated but many ethical problems lie in the way. The perfect approach would be to be able to encourage the patient's own tissues to reform lost organs. It may be that people will have their own tissue banks in future, from which organs may be grown at will.

Medicines are already and will increasingly become customized to particular patients, or at least groups of patients. It may be that people in a particular age group or with a particular genetic make up will be given a type of medication suited to that make up.

The continuing development of monoclonal antibodies is likely to be especially useful. These antibodies are substances produced from the culture of living tissues. They have a very long life and are produced by fusing together an antibody-forming white cell, known as a lymphocyte, with a tumour cell.[37] The antibody can be made specifically to react with a particular protein and can therefore be made to seek out abnormal cells. They link with suspicious cells in the body of a patient and help to diagnose what problem the patient is suffering from, or may even, in future, be used to destroy the abnormal cells. The antibodies, if they contain small amounts of radioactive material can be detected and used for outlining abnormal tissues without surgery. Abnormal cells, for instance cancer cells or blood vessels which are blocked, can be traced using this method.

One difficulty of increasing customization for medicines is a financial one. If a particular treatment is developed these days it requires considerable testing to ensure that it is safe and efficacious. This tends to make drug development expensive. These costs are recouped by selling the drug to many people. If drugs are customized they can, by definition be tested on and used for relatively small groups of people. It may well be that these treatments will be effective but too expensive for the pharmaceutical firms to think of developing.

▲ 83 How do these advances fit in with the problems that the NHS faces?

The depressing part about all of this is that the major advances appear to be in areas that are simply logical extensions of the old routines. The 'health' service is still obsessed with trying to patch up badly damaged bodies. The patching becomes steadily more technologically perfect, but we know that treating people late in life with one dread disease will mean that they will shortly present again with another. Most of the common diseases in developed countries such as heart disease, cancers and stroke, rapidly increase in likelihood during the later stages of life. As these different diseases behave similarly to each other, the likelihood of suffering more than one also increases with age.

In a number of international comparisons between causes of death it has been found that there was 'competition' for mortality between different diseases. For instance, stomach cancer and breast cancer in women showed a close relationship, as one increased the other decreased. The same held for breast cancer and tuberculosis. Similar interactions meant that there was little relationship between single causes of death and mortality from all causes. For instance, the contribution of death from cirrhosis of the liver to total mortality is completely compensated for by the effect of other causes of death. Thus if any one cause of death is reduced, it is possible, at least for some causes, that it will have little or no effect upon all deaths.[38]

It is important that we in the NHS learn the important lessons from these findings. A sensible approach to the prevention of disease is likely to be much more effective than following these logical progressions in medical practice to their illogical conclusions. There is enough effective preventative work to make an important difference to the effect medicine has, especially on relieving fear.

Approaches that are likely to be most effective are in carefully chosen screening programmes, the prevention of smoking and high immunization rates. The hard part will be having the courage to say no to extensions of the traditional approaches in order to divert, say, 10% of the NHS budget to the effective but less glamorous areas of work. Much of this indeed is outside the NHS altogether. The NHS may have to face the ultimate degree of altruism, to allow its budget to be taken over by education or housing or even to reduce public spending to allow the development of industries in poorer parts of the country.

▲ 84 What management changes are likely in the NHS?

At the time of writing, the NHS is going through yet another management-orientated reorganization. The provider trusts are being made into larger units and purchasing is to be centred on groups of GP-based purchasers for populations of about 100 000, with the health authorities assisting in their development. It seems likely that health authorities will be brought together in regional groups in the future. The simplest way of doing this would be to remove the health authority tier altogether, leaving the regions, which are branches of central government to oversee 20 to 30 GP-led purchasing groups. The government would then have very powerful control over the purchasing groups.

In this scenario, the purchasers would be smaller than the providers. The GPs may appear to hold the whip hand, as they could demand to purchase services from the provider trusts. However, the very large trusts could make life very uncomfortable for any one purchasing group if the only other option was to use a trust some distance away. The government has suggested that co-operation between the different parts of the health service will avoid such problems. In a world where everyone believes devoutly that he or she can do more good if they have more money and where there is a finite amount of cash, co-operation may not be enough.

▲ 85 How much will we spend on the NHS?

It is a truism to say that the demands on health services, especially if they are provided free at the point of access, as in the UK, are always greater than the supply.[39] There is a belief that society will not make difficult choices between demands for the money available, although this may be a perception of politicians wishing to run for election, who do not wish to pose the question for fear of the answer they will get.

Some years ago, a sample survey of over 4000 people aged 17 and over in Cardiff did pose some relevant questions.[40] People were told how much was spent on the main services provided by the government. Each pound of tax revenue was divided up between the main government-funded services. The people in the survey were asked in what way they would change the allocation, still keeping within the total of one pound sterling.

Figure 7.1 shows the results for people of different ages, compared with the amount allocated to the different services at the time. The public wanted more spent on health, education, housing, the environment and transport and wanted the money to be taken from social security, to some extent, and to a greater degree from defence. People felt that the greatest redistribution should be from defence services into health services.

The age groups were generally in agreement about which services should receive more, which should get less, but younger people were more radical in the degree of change that they suggested.

At the present time it seems inevitable that the total will continue to rise. Figure 7.2 shows that changes in the internal market approach resulted in more capital charges being included in the costs of the NHS, hence the recent rapid rise. The Labour government may try to reverse this, but the basic increase in wages year on year remains.

▲ 86 Why does health care cost so much?

Health care is expensive because it is labour intensive. Figure 7.2 shows the proportion of the NHS spent on salaries and wages since 1975. It can be seen that until 1991 about 75% of the costs of the health service was spent on these. After 1991 the government brought in capital charges and depreciation costs in order to ensure that the internal market would not work against the interests of private suppliers who had to meet such costs. There was also much more purchasing of services from non-NHS suppliers after that time. Salaries still remain the largest part of the costs of the NHS.

I have mentioned that the single largest section of the budget is on nurses' salaries. The numbers employed by the NHS have also

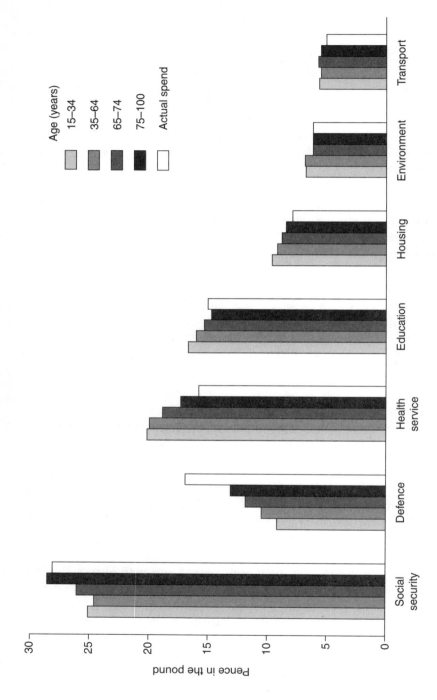

Figure 7.1: Public preferences for public expenditure.

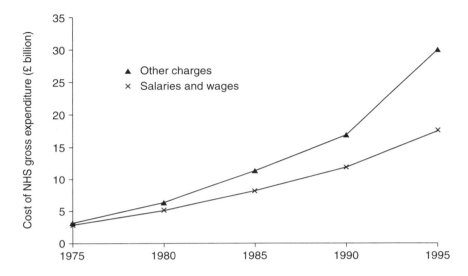

Figure 7.2: Gross expenditure on the NHS by salaries and other charges.

increased year on year since its inception until 1993, when numbers began to fall. This compares with education where the peak of employment was in 1988, with considerable falls since then.

There are also internal pressures in any health system for its costs to inflate. Specialists are, by tradition, given a wide range of power to decide on what to give their patients and in what circumstances. This is a competitive business. One specialist will wish to outdo other specialists in the equipment and the services they consume. New specialties are developing constantly. Oncologists were rare in the UK until recently. They are beginning to increase rapidly in number. In addition there is always pressure for greater safety; this increases the professionalisation of minor workers and thus increases their wages and the costs of the NHS.

The NHS is much more interventionist than it was in the past. Figure 7.3 shows the increases in the proportion of people admitted to hospital between 1968 and 1985. It can be seen that the proportion of admissions rose dramatically for all age groups, but especially

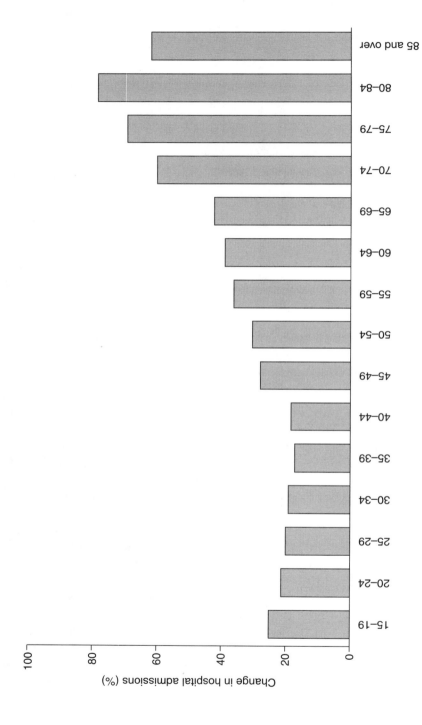

Figure 7.3: Change in hospital admissions per 1000 population, 1968–85.

those of retirement age. Part of this increase simply reflects that more people were in these age groups in 1985 than in 1968. The main reason for admission fell into the category of symptoms and signs, often used to categorize people with no obvious single disease but with marked social problems not allowing them to stay at home or with multiple disease problems. The problems of treating people with multiple diagnoses has already been mentioned above.

▲ 87 Do more doctors and nurses mean that people are healthier?

Archie Cochrane examined this question for developed countries. His work suggested that more doctors actually meant a higher infant mortality rate, usually taken to be an important measure of the health of a country.[41] I have looked again at some of these figures for the developed countries. If we compare the number of doctors available in countries that belong to the Organization of Economic Co-operation and Development (OECD) with the infant mortality rate as a measure of health the data appear as in Figure 7.4. The first thing that this figure shows is that countries have a great variation in the number of doctors per head, from 1 to 3.5 per 1000 population. This is a considerable difference for countries which are essentially at similar levels of development. The next thing that the figure shows is that there is no relationship between the number of doctors and the infant mortality rate. This is at least better than in the Cochrane paper, where more doctors were present in countries with the *worst* infant mortalities.

Nurses show up a little better than doctors. Figure 7.5 shows similar data to Figure 7.4 but for nurses. Once again there is a marked difference between countries in the number of nurses they employ but more nurses do seem to be present in countries with the best infant mortality rates. It is interesting that the relationship becomes much less obvious in those countries with more than five nurses

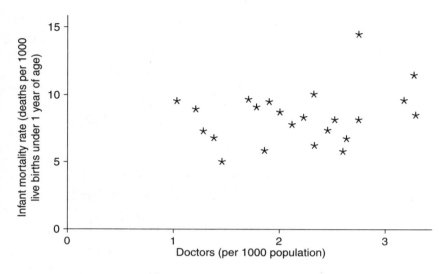

Figure 7.4: Relationship between number of doctors and infant mortality rate: OECD countries.

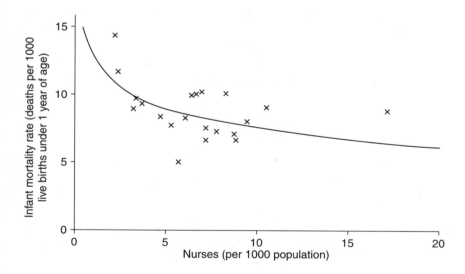

Figure 7.5: Relationship between number of nurses and infant mortality rate: OECD countries.

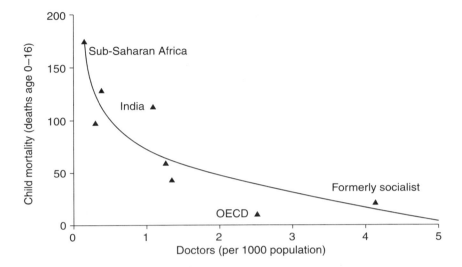

Figure 7.6: Relationship between child mortality and number of doctors (world groupings, 1990).

per 1000 population, suggesting that any more than that are superfluous.

These figures were for developed countries. Developing countries show a much more marked relationship between the number of doctors and nurses and their mortality rates. Figure 7.6 shows the data for doctors and infant mortality rate world-wide. However, the fact that doctors are more common in places with lower infant mortality rates may simply reflect the fact that they, as Illich says 'tend to gather where the climate is healthy, where the water is clean and where people are employed and can pay for their services.'[29]

▲ 88 How does NHS spending compare with other countries' health services?

I have shown that the wealth of a country relates to the health indices for that country. Given the amount spent on the NHS (about 6% of our gross domestic product in 1995) we seem to do fairly well in our health indices compared with our wealth as a country. The rate of increase in the costs of the health service has been rising fast during the 1990s compared with the 1960s and 1970s. The main contrast between the UK NHS and other countries is that the private sector for health care is very small in the UK.

In terms of value for money, Figure 7.7 shows the GDP per person against the infant mortality rate. The UK is on the line showing the relationship. This suggests that we are not especially cheap or costly

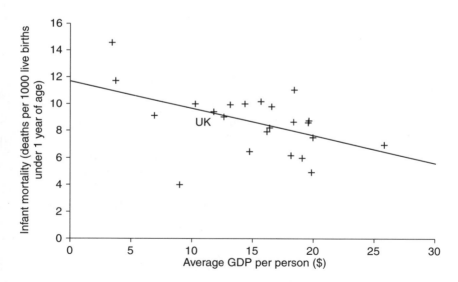

Figure 7.7: Relationship between GDP per person ($) and infant mortality rate: OECD countries.

compared with other OECD countries. In terms of infant mortality rate we are a little above half way. However, I have already suggested that infant mortality rate relates to overall spending, or the wealth of a country, but not as closely to health care spending.

▲ 89 How will the country answer the problems of health being mainly affected by factors other than health care?

I have tried to show throughout this book that health is much more affected by factors outside the control of the NHS than elements within it. The main known promoter of health in the UK is increasing personal wealth. The tendency for governments to avoid using public spending as a tool for improving wealth means that the best chance for improved health at a national level is to provide employment, especially for the poorest members of society. Over the last 20 years or so parts of the Welfare State, notably cheap housing, have been heavily undermined. This must have had a considerable and adverse effect upon health, a little of which has been obvious from the increasing inequalities in health in the UK during that time. The most extreme group of those affected by a reduction in cheap housing, the homeless, are known to suffer high levels of disease prevalence, from TB to musculo-skeletal, skin problems, infectious diseases and accidents. Those who are not on the streets but in temporary accommodation often have inadequate provision of food, drinking water and cooking facilities.[42]

The health of people is, of course, affected by much more than the things provided by the Welfare State. The problem with most of these things, such as diet, clothing and leisure activities, is that they depend heavily upon the amount of money the individual has and the other demands made upon it. Our consumption of things that

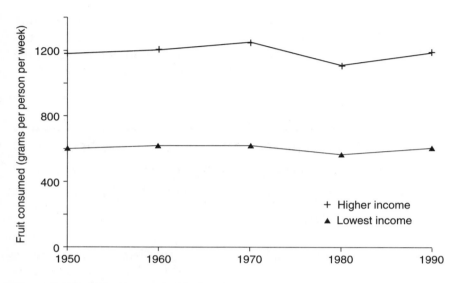

Figure 7.8: Fresh fruit consumed by income group.

everyone agrees are good for health, such as fresh fruit and vegetables, has grown greatly since the advent of the NHS,[43] but there
remains a marked difference between lower and higher income
groups (Figure 7.8).

▲ 90 How will the NHS deal with problems of communication?

I am concerned about the problem of the general public having a say
in the way that health services develop. In the UK, at present, the
most effective way is to depose the government of the day, and
therefore the Secretary of State, in a general election. This is hardly a
flexible way to bring about change. In the mean time it is to be hoped
that the purchasers of health services will take seriously the need to

be aware of what the general public wants and to be able to modify their plans, to some extent, towards those desires.

The work must be much more positive than simply asking the local population what they want. The issues are often complex and technical and will need to be translated into understandable choices, without paternalism or propaganda. This needs skill in communication and openness on the part of the NHS, which has not been an obvious part of its make up in the past. Most health authorities have attempted to get the views of the public or their patients about their plans in some way or another. However, vital questions are not asked, such as what values the local public hold, whether they prefer equality of access to high-powered centralized facilities, whether some treatment services should be disadvantaged for the development of preventative services in future.

It is essential that good straightforward non-propagandist information should be given to people to make sense of health issues. It is a failing of my own profession, public health medicine, that we have not taken on that task despite being well placed to do so. Maybe in the next few years we will be forced to take up this important work by government policy. If we do not do so, it is to be hoped that other groups will.

▲ 91 What is the future for primary care?

The 1978 Alma Ata declaration reinforced the importance of primary health care as the basis for diagnosis and treatment in both developing and developed countries.[44] Partly in response to that and partly because of parallel pressures to those felt in developed countries, a number of developing countries have been concentrating their money on primary care services. This has often entailed transferring clinical activities from the wards, operating theatres and special units in hospital to local outpatient departments, day care units and home and community-based services. This diversion of effort has also involved a strong health promotion aspect. In a book on the subject, Paine makes the central point: 'Such actions are beginning to break through the carapace of assured self-containment with which many of the highly skilled, highly qualified professional staff of the hospital have too often surrounded themselves in the past.'[45]

These ideas were not new. Paine describes a 'hospital without walls' programme set up 30 years before in Costa Rica despite considerable governmental and other opposition. The hospital still acts as a co-ordinating point for five health centres, five social security clinics and 46 health posts distributed throughout the area which it serves. It helps to develop health education and training for professionals in the community. A similar approach has been used in Nepal where a small district hospital is the central point for a large community organization. Health posts manned by paramedical staff serve the local population. The hospital resolutely refuses to develop tertiary or sub-specialty services, preferring to use its energy to develop further the primary care facilities scattered around it.

Such approaches are not confined to developing countries. The North Central Bronx Hospital in New York facing similar problems of large numbers of deprived people in the area set up a Neighbourhood Family Care Centre in 1973, which attempted to treat families rather than disease. Specialist clinics in the hospital were phased out and replaced by five primary health care teams acting as independent units and responsible for all of the care for a particular group of families in the district. These teams included junior doctors, nurse practitioners, social workers, community nurses and family health technicians.[46] In another example, in Bihar, a particularly poor area of India, the only family hospital has 14 departments, one of which is run by a graduate of the College of Agriculture so that the health promotion message includes ways of improving agricultural efficiency.

It seems that in poor areas, where it is obvious that the main causes of ill health are social and therefore require social answers, the health service is forced to break down its walls in order to provide social answers. There have been suggestions that the developed world could benefit from these ideas more generally to help to meet increasing financial demands.

▲ 92 How has primary care failed in the NHS?

The GPs were not very convinced about the usefulness of the NHS from its outset and the vast majority still holds it at arm's length by being independent contractors. It may be argued that, at least for the first 40 years, they were right. They were the second class citizens. Partly as a result, any vital point in the history of the NHS, when major changes have been about to occur, the GPs, or at least a reasonably large number of them, threaten not to renew their contracts. Salaried GPs are still a rarity, although recent suggestions from the government about 'Primary Care Trusts' suggest that salaried GPs may be about to be tried on a wider scale.

Primary care, especially for GPs, has had enormous opportunities, most of which it has, with honourable exceptions, avoided. The opportunities lie in two areas: prevention of disease and countering inequity between the rich and the poor. General practices have been in a perfect position to work on both of these problems, but instead have concentrated on treating minor diseases with largely ineffective treatment. Again it has not entirely been their fault. In the early days of the NHS they were not allowed to stray from the treatment path, but more recently with changes in the GP contract and fundholding they could have taken over the whole area. The greatest loss has been advice to people about cigarette smoking. The most effective way of getting someone to stop smoking is to be told to do so by your own GP. The opportunity is rarely taken, with important exceptions.[47]

When GPs do it, they are good at presentation. Figure 7.9 shows data for an area just outside Cardiff, where breast and cervical screening are carried out. Breast screening is performed centrally, cervical

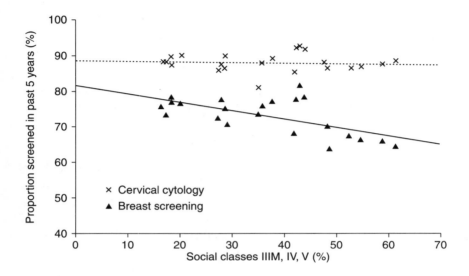

Figure 7.9: Relationship between screening and social class by electoral ward in the Vale of Glamorgan.

screening by the GPs. It can be seen that the GPs cover the poor areas of the patch much more effectively than the centrally run breast screening.

▲ 93 How will the NHS try to deal with poor communication, both personal and organizational?

Dr Halfdan Mahler, a previous Director General of the World Health Organization (WHO), has suggested that medicine had progressively, whether consciously or unconsciously, set up a 'mystification of medical care'. He mentioned that, in order to maintain this mystification, the specialties continue to restrict the range of problems that they consider themselves responsible for. He stated that the gap between the maintenance of health care and medical care is becoming increasingly wider.

He also described the restrictions set up on the information available about health care. Decisions that have been made by people in the health professions mean that the general population has become increasingly dependent upon the holders of these mysteries. Dr Mahler suggested that it is the job of people in public health medicine who are the heirs of the great men of 19th century public health to become, like them, social reformers. Their first job is to free the public from the mysteries, by explaining them in detail and then to point out the extreme importance of other, more politically sensitive, social conditions such as housing, unemployment and poverty on the health of groups and individuals within those groups.

Dr Mahler describes the gross inequality in health expenditure in developing countries, which, in contrast to the past, is no longer spent on the wealthy but on an equally small proportion of the population which medical technology defines itself as being capable of dealing with. He mentions that this expenditure has never been proved to increase life expectancy or to improve the last few years of life. Despite this, most of the expenditure occurs during this last period of existence. There appears to be a trend towards defining the 'best' health care as where everything known to medicine is applied to every individual by the highest trained medical scientist in the most specialized institution.

In the 20 years since Dr Mahler wrote his article there has been some reaction against the mystification of health. There have been attempts made to give people more knowledge of the origins of disease beyond simple ideas of germ theory and hygiene. For example, almost everyone in developed countries knows that smoking is bad for health. However there is little idea, for instance, of the relative impact of cigarettes or the motor car upon our health. In rare cases difficult decisions about what to do with scarce health money has been the subject of carefully organized wide public debate but this is very rare and, as the people of Oregon discovered, expensive and fraught with political pitfalls.[49]

There is some, although not much, questioning of the place of the super specialties in improving health. Cardiac transplantation, for instance, was questioned about its effectiveness when many of the early cases died, but as more individuals survived the fuss subsided. There is little questioning about the central philosophy of developing such expensive treatments for such small numbers of people or the right of the bio-engineering and medical professions to develop such approaches as long as they appear to work at a technical level.

▲ 94 How will the NHS deal with inequity?

The main problem appears to be getting good NHS services to poor people. I have mentioned the non-NHS problems, but within the NHS there are marginal improvements that one can make to improve the access of poor people to the NHS. It may be that, with the new Primary Care Groups as commissioning bodies, we need to provide a set of core services but with new ideas being tried out in different places, depending upon the nature of the specific problems in that area. By their nature, local services are small-scale and therefore can take risks with the type of service that each provides. They are able to aim at sub-groups, who might normally receive little attention, such as ethnic groups, homeless people, mobile families, homosexuals. Institutions appear to be much less helpful to people in inner cities than in other places. However, the same argument would apply to any community which had unusual problems. Indeed, it may be said that all small communities have special characteristics and that primary and community services should be tailored to those peculiarities.

A number of possible answers to these problems have been suggested in the past. Examples have been sick bays for homeless and indigent people, the use of salaried GPs where the population is constantly changing, specialist community nurses for families in bed and breakfast accommodation. It has been suggested that there should be interpretation and advocacy services for people in ethnic minorities, outreach teams for people who are misusing drugs and those living on the streets or in hostels. Other suggestions have included ambulatory care centres where a range of walk-in services is available including specialist clinics, diagnostic facilities and minor surgery. These approaches have all been tried out piecemeal, but are poorly evaluated and remain isolated ideas.

Community nurses in particular will have to work in a number of innovative ways, some of which they may find restrictive as they will be working, unusually, directly with consultants. A similar move towards the planning and delivery of services in small populations may now be possible if the Primary Care Groups decide to work in this way.

▲ 95 How will the NHS deal with rising costs?

We have two consolations about health spending in the UK. First, it is not as bad as in some places and second, everyone else is worrying about it. It has been said that two major factors have kept down the costs in the NHS: the GP gatekeeper system and our tendency not to pay our professionals very much in comparison with other countries. It is obvious that, if we want to keep a fairly cheap service, we need to protect both of these.

Small improvements can be made to the service by keeping efficiency high. This will mean a close look at the way that clinical services are run, for non-clinical services have been assessed and retested many times. In particular, this will mean close management control over what professionals do. This is not a cheerful message for the health service, where the battle between managers and doctors is swinging the doctors' way since the Labour government came to power. It has not been possible in the past for managers to take on the might of the clinicians on their own ground. Many managers in battles with consultants have lost their jobs, and government departments and health authorities have rarely intervened on the managers' behalf.

Some people hold out hopes for keeping costs down by appealing directly to professionals by pressing for only clinically effective treatment to be used. This may help to hold down some outlandish proposals, but it is a blunt instrument. Governments hope that, because so few medical interventions have solid scientific evidence for them, there will be pressure on specialists to reduce the number of interventions undertaken. However, the clinical effectiveness approach always leaves the door open for an individual professional with an individual patient to try anything reasonable. The basis of this is that human beings vary so greatly that, on occasion, unusual remedies may work. This is a fact. Scientific evidence, as mentioned above, is based on the analysis of averages. But not all humans are average. As a cost-saving exercise, clinical effectiveness is likely to be a non-starter.

8

Conclusion: has it worked?

▲ 96 What else is the NHS for?

The Guillebaud committee in 1953 stated that: 'In the absence of an objective and attainable standard of adequacy, the aim must be ... to provide the best service possible within the limits of the available resources.' Bevan believed that it was there to relieve fear. I have tried to show ways in which the NHS has, in the past failed to do that. The close relatives of fear are ignorance and pain. The NHS has not been very good at removing either over the years, not from lack of technical knowledge in the subjects, but because it did not realize the importance of these things. The management of a connected fear, that of death, has developed by leaps and bounds in the past ten years; largely by pressure from outside the health service. While these services for the care of the dying have been progressing, they have also given us more skills in the prevention of pain and the need to take it more seriously.

▲ 97 Has the NHS been too slow to change?

People often say that the NHS is slow to change. The NHS is an organization that costs £40 billion a year, with management costs of about 6% of the total. I believe that, given this, the people in the organization have shown the most amazing adaptability over the past 25 years. The management costs compare favourably with British Rail, which, before privatization, had costs of about 12%. There have been problems. There were instances in the early days of the internal market where the purchasers and providers were dealing in different measures in the contract. I have seen examples where one group believed the contract to be measured in the number of patients seen (discharges and deaths). The other based the contract on the number of days patients were in hospital (bed-days). Considerable confusion followed when the bills came in.

The one thing managers have been reluctant to do is to suggest improvements to the efficiency of the bulk of the work, the clinical services. The few managers who have attempted to change clinical services have usually come a cropper. Doctors, nurses and therapists have a tendency to refuse to listen if a 'lay' person attempts to change their practice by even a tiny amount. Clinical audit, which was supposed, at least, to bring the worst offenders up to the average, is slow to have an effect.

▲ 98 Why have there been so many changes in the NHS?

The good, or maybe bad, news about all the UK changes is that no other country is satisfied with its health system. There appear to be four types of problem (Box 8.1).

Box 8.1 Problems with health services internationally

- **Finance.** Every developed country thinks it pays too much for its health service and that the payment is increasingly getting out of control. The USA has managed to develop a system of high administrative costs with low control over the service. The UK by contrast has low administrative costs and a high degree of control. Most other countries fall between these two extremes, but none are happy about the amount they spend.
- **Delivery of services.** All developed countries seem to have doubts about the quality or the access of patients to their services. Poor people do not, even when the service is free at the point of delivery, have equal access to services.
- **Efficiency.** There is a common belief that all health services can be made more efficient. This leads to more central control of the way services are provided. Recently this has led to the use of guidelines and detailed descriptions of how we should provide health care, intended to allow managers more control over the clinicians. Governments have ostensibly brought about these changes to improve the effectiveness of care. There may be an antipathy between efficiency and effectiveness, which most governments feign not to appreciate.
- **Limits to health care.** Some believe that redefining what the health service provides will clarify what they are trying to do. This ranges from a belief in more prevention and health promotion, through taking personal responsibility for one's health, to restricting health care to the acute treatment of diseases which have effective treatment.

Several examples of the problem in defining health care have arisen in the NHS. One was a row about whether the health service should provide some or no continuing care for elderly people. Others have included arguments about whether the treatment of scars, other forms of cosmetic surgery and assisted fertilization services should be provided on the NHS. Some people believed that these things are not what health care is about.

In regard to the relation between health and social services, I have enjoyed much hilarity in committees between health and social services people trying to decide if health or social services should provide bathing for elderly people. Several answers came up, ranging from the mundane (it should be health if they are dirty, social if they are clean) to the risqué (health if they are alone, social if with company). The two are, of course, inextricably linked. Administrative lines can be drawn, but they make no intrinsic sense.

▲ 99 Has the NHS been good for equity?

There is little doubt, but no direct evidence, that the NHS ensured that everyone in the UK was able to get access to a group of fully trained specialists within about 10 years of setting up the NHS. Everyone was also put onto the list of a GP within months of the NHS starting. The quality of these doctors was higher in well-to-do areas and in the not-too-bleak country areas than in the centre of cities and the industrial wastelands of, for instance Lancashire and South Wales. These differences remain today and have been very difficult to eradicate. The latest attempt to do so in London, in response to the Tomlinson Report, is still having difficulty in being fully implemented.[49]

Equity of outcome, of deaths and disabilities, have not reduced as a result of the NHS, as a recent major publication on inequalities in health has shown.[33] For almost every group of diseases the difference between rich and poor has been maintained; if anything it has been widening.

▲ 100 Has the NHS relieved fear?

The general population welcomed the setting up of the NHS in 1948 with open arms. It has remained a favourite with the public ever since. The British social attitudes survey has been asking people what they think of the health service since 1983. It consistently shows very high levels of satisfaction with the NHS. Women consistently report higher levels of satisfaction than men.

Satisfaction with GPs is consistently greater than with the rest of the NHS. There has been little change in this degree of satisfaction with the GPs over the years. The researchers asked people what improvements to the services they would suggest. The main problem that patients had with GPs was the appointment system. Four out of ten people recommended some change. As far as hospital services were concerned most people were satisfied with the quality of medical treatment, especially nursing care, but waiting times for non-emergency operations caused considerable concern. There was also some concern about the physical layout of hospitals.

There was a marked change over the years in answer to a question about whether the government should increase taxes so that spending on health, education and social benefits could be improved. Between 1983 and 1993, double the percentage of people, from a third to two-thirds, thought that increased taxes should be spent. Interestingly, during this period, people had voted for the political party that promised to cut taxes.

On a more personal note, individual patients still have concerns about their own treatment. In contrast with many other developed countries and most developing countries, fear of not being able to afford treatment is not a problem, as a result of the NHS. In some ways NHS treatment is superior to treatment in the private sector in the UK. The large number of people in training in the NHS ensures a better staffing ratio and emergency cover than in most private hospitals.

The main areas of failure to relieve fear are fears relating to ignorance, pain and death. The NHS, with varying degrees of success, is addressing the last two. Ignorance is still rife. This is not simply a UK problem but the NHS has a number of attributes which make it worse (Box 8.2) The international problems of doctors and patients finding it hard to talk to each other have been outlined above.

These problems are not insurmountable, they are simply not addressed as a central part of what the organization is trying to achieve. My belief is that these are not peripheral issues, but central to the way that the NHS must progress.

Box 8.2 Problems remaining in the NHS

- There is still a slight feeling that the NHS is the second tier service. 'If you want to be called by your second name go to BUPA, the private health care service' (overheard on a hospital ward).
- The relationship between service given and payment received is not obvious to professionals.
- The NHS is very big. Patients often see different people each time they use the service. It is difficult to have a personal relationship, even with GPs.

▲ 101 How can this be summarized?

The greatest known danger to health, apart from poverty and its effects, is poor nutrition and something best described by a word that Beveridge would recognize: hopelessness. We can easily forget that the five giants – want, ignorance, squalor, idleness and disease – are all part of the same whole. The Welfare State was set up as a spectrum of services for helping people and the spectrum merges imperceptibly between each colour. It is meaningless to spare the NHS but attack other segments of the Welfare State. Health suffers from poverty and unemployment, but also from lack of housing, education and social services. It probably suffers least, in terms of mortality and morbidity at a national level, from cuts to the NHS. Cuts to the NHS do, however, engender fear in people who do, or may, need to use the service. It is the main job of the NHS to relieve that fear.

References

1 DoH (1991) *The health of the nation* (Cmnd 1523). HMSO, London.

2 Gosbee J (1998) Communication among health professionals (editorial). *BMJ.* **318**: 642.

3 Salvage AV (1986) *Attitudes of the over-75s to health and social services.* Research Team for the Care of the Elderly, Cardiff.

4 Borough of Hackney (1985) *A study of the awareness of Haringey residents of the Social Services Department and general attitudes towards social services.* Social Services Department, London Borough of Haringey.

5 British Medical Association (1977) *You and your baby.* Family Doctor Publications, BMA, London.

6 Cay EL, Vetter NJ, Philip AE *et al.* (1973) Return to work after a heart attack. *J Psychosomatic Research.* **17**: 231–43.

7 Bentall RP (1992) A proposal to classify happiness as a psychiatric disorder. *J Medical Ethics.* **18**: 94–8.

8 Halstead SB, Walsh JA and Warren KS (1983) *Good health at low cost.* Rockefeller Foundation, New York.

9 Tudor Hart J (1971) The inverse care law. *Lancet.* **1**: 405–12.

10 Payer L (1988) *Medicine and culture.* Viking Penguin, New York.

11 Silverman WA (1993) Doing more harm than good. In WA Warren and F Mosteller (eds) Doing more harm than good. *Annals of New York Academy of Sciences.* **703**: 5–11.

12 Beveridge Report (1942) *Social insurance and allied services* (Cmnd 6404). HMSO, London.

13 Hasler J (1992) The primary health care team: history and contractual farces. *BMJ.* **305**: 232–4.

14 Editorial (1958) *BMJ.* **Suppl 1**: 27.

15 Smith JW and Mottram EM (1967) Extended use of nursing services in general practice. *BMJ.* **4**: 672–4.

16 Ministry of Health (1962) *A hospital plan for England and Wales* (Cmnd 1604). HMSO, London.

17 Committee on Child Health Services (1976) *Fit for the future: report of the Committee on Child Health Services* (Cmnd 6684). HMSO, London.

18 Cochrane AL (1971) *Effectiveness and efficiency: random reflections on the health service.* Nuffield Provincial Hospitals Trust, London.

19 Wolfensberger W (1972) *The principle of normalisation in human services.* National Institute on Mental Retardation, Toronto.

20 Levin E, Sinclair IA and Gorbach P (1989) *Families, services and confusion in old age.* Gower, Aldershot.

21 DHSS (1983) *The Griffith Report: NHS management inquiry.* DHSS, London.

22 Fowler N (1991) *Ministers decide: a personal memoir of the Thatcher years.* Chapman & Hall, London.

23 Butler J (1994) Origins and early development. In R Robinson and J Le Grand (eds) *Evaluating the NHS reform.* King's Fund Institute, London.

24 DHSS (1983) *Competitive tendering in the provision of domestic catering and laundry services* (HC (83) 18). DHSS, London.

25 Houseman S, Hunter D and Pollit C (1990) *The dynamics of British health policy.* Unwin Hyman, London.

26 Enthoven AC (1985) *Reflections on the management of the NHS*. Occasional Paper 5. Nuffield Provincial Hospitals Trust, London.

27 Binstock RH and Post SG (eds) (1991) *Too old for health care: controversies in medicine, law, economics and ethics*. Johns Hopkins University Press, Baltimore.

28 Kennedy I (1981) *The unmasking of medicine*. Allen and Unwin, London.

29 Illich I (1977) *Limits to medicine*. Penguin Books, London.

30 McKeown T (1977) *The role of medicine*. Blackwell, London.

31 Phillipp R, Hughes A, Wood N *et al.* (1990) Information needs of patients and visitors in a district general hospital. *J Royal Society of Health*. **1**: 10–12.

32 Black D (1982) *Inequalities in health*. Penguin, Harmondsworth.

33 Drewer F and Whitehead M (1997) *Health inequalities*. Government Statistical Service, London.

34 DoH (1989) *Self-governing hospitals* (Working paper No 1). HMSO, London.

35 Abel-Smith B (1964) *The hospitals, 1800–1948*. Heinemann, London.

36 Education Committee (1993) *Recommendations on undergraduate medical training*. General Medical Council, London.

37 Office of Technology Assessment (1984) *Commercial biotechnology: an international analysis*. US Government Printing Office, Washington DC.

38 Gavrilov LA and Gavrilova NS (1991) *The biology of life span: a quantitative approach*. Harwood Academic Publishers, Switzerland.

39 Blank RH (1991) Rationing medicine: hard choices in the 1990s. *American J Gastroenterology*. **87**: 1076–84.

40 Charney MS, Lewis PA and Farrow SC (1989) Choosing who shall not be treated in the NHS. *Social Science and Medicine*. **28**: 1331–8.

41 Cochrane AL (1975) World health problems. *Canadian J Public Health*. **66**: 280–5.

42 Charlton J and Murphy M (eds) *The health of adult Britain (Vol 1)*. Office for National Statistics, London.

43 MAFF (1991) *Household food consumption and expenditure, 1990.* HMSO, London.

44 World Health Organisation (1978) *Primary health care. Alma Ata, Health for All Series, No 1.* WHO, Geneva.

45 Paine LH and Siem Tjam F (1988) *Hospitals and the health care revolution.* WHO, Geneva.

46 Macagba R (1985) *Hospitals and primary health care.* International Hospital Federation, London.

47 Tudor Hart J (1981) A new kind of doctor. *J Royal Society of Medicine.* **74**: 871–83.

48 Klein R (1991) On the Oregon trail. *BMJ.* **302**: 1–2.

49 DoH (1993) *The Tomlinson Report. Making London better.* DoH, London.

Index

1940s 20–35
1950s 36–48
1960s 36–48
1970s 49–60
1980s 61–74
1990s 75–93
2000s 94–116

administrative changes 50–1, 63–4
admissions *see* hospitals
air pollution reductions 40
alternative therapy 19
Area Health Authorities 50
Area Medical Committees 51

Bevan, Aneurin 7, 31–2
Beveridge, Sir William 26
Beveridge Report 26
    response to 27
        GPs 29
        hospitals 27–8
Black, Sir Douglas 72–3, 91
BMA *see* British Medical Association

Bosanquet, Nick 74
British Hospitals Association 27
British Medical Association (BMA)
    GPs' disgust with 41
    GPs' reaction to NHS 32–3
    health policy 69

Castle, Barbara 54
child mortality
    and numbers of doctors *105*
    see also infant mortality rate
Clarke, Kenneth 74
clinical effectiveness 56, 80
    and cost-saving 116
    definition *80*
    increased interest in *81*
Cochrane, Archie 55–6, 80, 103
commissioning groups 84
communication
    doctors and patients 71–2
    health services problems 35
    NHS 46, 55–6, 69–72, 89–90, 108–9
    personal and organizational 112–14

community health clinics 44
community medicine 51
community nurses 114–15
community staff 42–3
competition 67
competitive tendering 65
consensus management 50, 54
contracting out clinical services 65
Cost Rent Scheme 62
costs
    of health care 99–103
    inflation pressures 101
    internal market 86
    rising
        health services problems 35
        NHS 47–8, 58–60, 73–4, 92–3,
        115–16
Court Report 53
customization of medicines 95–6

data revolution 94–5
death and disability
    avoidance, wealth of population
        relationships 15–16
    NHS
        lack of effects on 2–5
        reduction main aim 6–7
    reducing 5–6
death rates, publication 6–7
delivery of services problems 119
developed countries
    body of knowledge 18–19
    health services effects on health or
        disease 13
    infectious diseases, control 14
    primary care 109–10
    proportions of doctors and
        nurses to healthier people
        103–5, 104
developing countries
    health services effects on health or
        disease 13–14

proportions of doctors and nurses to
    healthier people 105
diminishing returns, law of 5
disability see death and disability
disabled people, benefits for 26
district general hospitals 44, 51, 52–3
district nurses 53

efficiency problems 119
Emergency Medical Service 24
employment, NHS 11
Enthoven, Alain 66–8, 73
environment, effects on individual
    health 14
equity of provision of health services
    35, 47, 57, 72–3, 90–1, 114–15, 120

Family Doctor's Charter 1966: 42
fear, relieving
    health services 1–2
    NHS 1–2, 7–9, 8
        failure to relieve 117, 121–2
        removing ignorance 10
        treatment of pain 9
finance problems 119
fundholding 74
    abolition 83
    internal market problems 86
    nature 82–3
    general managers 63–4

General Medical Council (GMC)
    communication concerns 89–90
general practice
    changes
        1950s and 1960s 41–2
        1970s 53
        1980s 62–3
        1990s 82–3
    nurses in 42, 62
general practitioners (GP)
    bad times in 1950s and 1960s 41–2

Beveridge Report, response to 29
community staff, relationship with
    42–3
Cost Rent Scheme 62
fundholding *see* fundholding
post-graduate training 62
purchasing groups 83
reaction to NHS 32–3
salaried 111
visiting before NHS 23
General Practitioners Association 41
geriatrics 38–9
GMC *see* General Medical Council
Godber, Sir George 51
GP *see* general practitioners
Griffiths, Sir Roy 63, 66
Guillebaud committee 36, 47–8, 117

health
  effects on *14*
  effects suffered from 122–3
  meaning 13
  NHS effect on 13–15
  non-NHS changes influencing in
    1950s and 1960s 40
health authorities
  boards 77
    selection 78–9
  health care
  expensiveness 99–103
  limits *119*
health care services
  effects on individual health *14*
health education groups 68, 88
health professionals and patients,
  relationship between 5
health promotion groups
  68–9, 88
health service data 12
health services
  problems faced *34*, 34–5
  internationally *119*

reasons for existence 18–19
relieving fear 1–2
health visitors 53
Hospital Management Committees 53
hospital medicine
  changes 1980s 61–2
  changes 1990s 79–82
Hospital Plan 1962: 43–4
  GPs 44
hospitals
  admissions 101–3, *102*
  and unemployment 11, *12*
  Beveridge Report, response to 27–8
  care before NHS 24–5
  development of 23–4
  length of stay variations in different
    countries *82*
  Regional Boards 43–4
  see also local authority hospitals;
    district general hospitals;
    voluntary hospitals
human biology, effects on individual
  health *14*

ignorance, removing 10
Illich, Ivan 70
incapacity for work 3, *4*
income generation schemes 65
inequity of provision of health services
  35, 47, 57, 72–3, 90–1, 114–15
infant mortality rate 2, *2*
  and gross domestic product *15*, *106*
  numbers of doctors and nurses
    and *104*
intensive treatment 49
internal market 67, 73, 75
  abolition 83
  costing emphasis 86
  developments leading to *65*
  fundholders, problems for 86
  position of 79
  pressure for change 76–7

providers 76, 79
purchasers 76, 79
strengths 84–5
weaknesses 85–7
International Classification of
    Diseases 18
Internet 94–5
inverse care law 17
    reasons for *17–18*

Kennedy, Ian 69–70

Labour government's changes 1997:
    83–4
law of diminishing returns 5
life expectancy
    at age 65: 3, *4*
    and gross domestic product *16*
    at birth 3, *3*
        different social classes *91*
lifestyle, effects on individual
    health *14*
Lloyd George, David 22
local authority hospitals 22, 23
    care 25
    integration with voluntary hospitals
        into NHS 24

Mahler, Halfdan 112–13
management changes 64–6, 97–8
Maynard, Alan 74
McColl, Ian 73–4
McKeown, Thomas 70
McKinzey report 50
Medical Officers of Health 42, 51, 52
Medical Practitioners Union 41
medical research, NHS support 12–13
medical schools 28
mentally handicapped and mentally ill
        people
    moving out of long-term hospital
        care 58

mystification of medical care
    112–13

National Health Service (NHS)
    changes
        in 1950s and 1960s 36–7
        reasons for 118–20
        slowness of 118
    communication 35, 46, 55–6, 69–72,
        89–90, 108–14
    costs, rising 35, 47–8, 58–60, 73–4,
        92–3, 115–16
    creation, reasons for 21–2
    death and disability
        lack of effects on 2–5
        reduction main aim 6–7
    death rates, publication 6–7
    effects on health other than by health
        service 34, 46, 54–5, 68–9, 88–9,
        107–8
    employment 11
    equal opportunities for all to benefit
        29–31
    equity of provision 35, 47, 57, 72–3,
        90–1, 114–15, 120
    expenditure and changes in political
        party 58–60, *59*
    funding and political party changes
        58–60, *59*
    governments, repeated
        reorganizations 87–8
    GPs' reaction to 32–3
    health, effect on 13–15
    health service data 12
    idea for 25–6
    inequity of provision 35, 47, 57, 72–3,
        90–1, 114–15
    management changes 64–6,
        97–8
    medical research support 12–13
    patients, differences for 33–4
    popular satisfaction with 121

problems
    advances and 96–7
    remaining 122
    relieving fear 1–2, 7–9, 8
        failure in 117, 121–2
        removing ignorance 10
        treatment of pain 9
    salaries and other charges 101
    spending on 98–9
        comparison with other countries
            106–7
    training function 12
National Insurance, manual workers 22
NHS see National Health Service
'ninepence for fourpence' system 22, 23
Nobel laureates of Britain 39, 40
nurses
    community 114–15
    district 114–15
    in general practice 42, 62
    salaries 99–101
    training 49–50

pain
    prevention 117
    treatment of, NHS 9
panel doctors 22
patients
    changes in 2000s 94–5
    and health professionals, relationship
        between 5
    ignorance 10
    knowledgeability, increasing 5
    NHS formation, differences on 33–4
    treatment available in 1940s 20–1
pay bargaining 93
payment for health services before
        NHS 22
political parties
    NHS funding and expenditure and
        58–60, 59
'polyclinics' 44

Poor Law hospitals 23
post-graduate training, GPs 62
practice of medicine, changes in
    1950s and 1960s 37–9
    1970s 49–50
prescription charges
    introduction of 44–5
    proportion of NHS total costs 45
primary care
    failure in NHS 111–12
    future for 109–11
Primary Care Groups 83, 114
Primary Care Trusts 83, 111
priority services 57–8
providers 76, 79
public health 89
public health medicine 113
public preferences for public
        expenditure 100
purchasers 76, 79

RCGP (Royal College of General
        Practitioners) 41
Regional Health Authorities 50
Regional Hospital Boards 43–4, 50, 53
Royal College of General Practitioners
        (RCGP) 41
Royal Colleges
    separation of physicians and
        surgeons 38

scientific changes 39–40, 95–6
scientific medicine 37–8
scientific research 39–40
screening, social class and 112
Seebohm report 52
smokeless zones 40
social answers 110
social class, screening and 112
social workers 52
Socialist Medical Association 25
specialist care growth 49

specialists 38
specialties 52–3

teaching hospitals 28
team management 50, 54
Thatcher, Margaret 64–6, 76–7, 87
Tomlinson Report 120
training
  GPs, post-graduate 62
  NHS function 12
  nurses 49–50
tripartite system removal 52
trusts 76
  boards 77
    selection 78–9

unemployment, and hospital
    admission 11, 12
Unit Managers 64

voluntary hospitals 21–2, 23
  charges 24
  free treatment 22
  integration with local
      authority hospitals into
      NHS 24

Warren, Marjory 39
wealth of population 15–16
welfare spending, 1921–91: 37
World Health Organization (WHO) 18